THE SPACE
BETWEEN OUR EARS

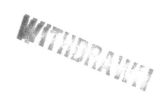

THE SPACE
BETWEEN OUR EARS

How the Brain Represents Visual Space

Michael Morgan

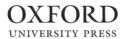

OXFORD
UNIVERSITY PRESS

OXFORD
UNIVERSITY PRESS

Great Clarendon Street, Oxford OX2 6DP

Oxford University Press is a department of the University of Oxford.
It furthers the University's objective of excellence in research, scholarship,
and education by publishing worldwide in

Oxford New York

Auckland Cape Town Dar es Salaam Hong Kong Karachi
Kuala Lumpur Madrid Melbourne Mexico City Nairobi
New Delhi Shanghai Taipei Toronto

With offices in

Argentina Austria Brazil Chile Czech Republic France Greece
Guatemala Hungary Italy Japan Poland Portugal Singapore
South Korea Switzerland Thailand Turkey Ukraine Vietnam

Oxford is a registered trade mark of Oxford University Press
in the UK and in certain other countries

Published in the United States
by Oxford University Press Inc., New York

British Library Cataloguing in Publication Data

Data available

Library of Congress Cataloging in Publication Data

Data available

Typeset by Selwood Systems, Midsomer Norton and
Newgen Imaging Systems (P) Ltd., Chennai, India
Printed in Great Britain
on acid-free paper by
Biddles Ltd, King's Lynn

ISBN 0–19–856955–6 978–0–19–856955–8

1 3 5 7 9 10 8 6 4 2

Contents

Figure Acknowledgments

Fig. 1.1 From Webster, M. A., Georgeson, M. A., & Webster, S. M. (2002). Neural adjustments to image blur. *Nat Neurosci, 5,* 839-842 with permission of the authors and Nature Publishing Group

Fig. 1.2 Copyright 2003 by Michael Morgan

Fig. 1.3 Thompson Thatcher Illusion, with permission

Fig. 1.4 From Linden, D. E., Kallenbach, U., Heinecke, A., Singer, W., & Goebel, R. (1999). The myth of upright vision. A psychophysical and functional imaging study of adaptation to inverting spectacles. *Perception, 28*(4), 469-481 with permission of the authors and Pion Limited

Fig. 2.1 With permission from Multimedia Library, Service Documentaire, Ecole Nationale des Ponts et Chaussées, Paris

Fig. 2.2 From Jacobson, M (1962) Quarterly Journal of Experimental Physiology, 47, 170-8 (Fig. 2) with permission of the Physiological Society

Fig. 3.1 From Glickstein, M & Fahle, M (2000) Brain Special Supplement Vol 123 Fig 5 and 38 with permission of the authors and Oxford University Press

Fig. 3.2 From Anstis, S. M. (1974). A chart demonstrating variations in acuity with retinal position. *Vision Research, 14,* 589-592 with permission from the author and Elsevier

Fig. 3.3 From Wiesel, T. Postnatal development of the visual cortex and the influence of environment. *Nature, 299,* 583-591 (Fig. 1) with permission of the author and Nature Publishing Group

Fig. 4.1 From p. 19 of M. Moss & I. Russell (1988) 'Range and Vision' Edinburgh: Mainstream Publishing with permission of Professor Michael Moss of Glasgow University

Fig. 4.2 From R.L. Gregory "Odd Perceptions" (Fig 11.8 on p. 74) with permission from Thompson Publishing Services

Fig. 4.3 Copyright 2003 by Michael Morgan

Fig. 4.4 From PhD thesis: Peter D Lunn (1994) The Perception of Stereoscopic Surfaces, Institute of Ophthalmology, UCL, with permission of the author

Fig. 5.1 Copyright Bayerisches National Museum, reproduced with permission

Fig. 5.2 Copyright 2003 by Michael Morgan

Fig. 5.3 Copyright 2003 by Michael Morgan; insert of Exner reproduced with permission of the Vienna Academy of Sciences

Fig. 6.1 From Plate 7 in J.T. Sumida (1989) In Defence of Naval Supremacy. Boston: Unwin Hyman, with permission of the MOD Admiralty Library

Fig. 6.2 Copyright Lucent Technologies Inc/ Bell Labs, reprinted with permission
Figs. 9.1–9.3 Copyright 2003 Michael Morgan
Fig. 9.4.1 Attneave's cat reproduced from Attneave, F. (1954). Some informational aspects of visual perception. *Psychological Review, 61(3)*, 183-193 with permission of the American Psychological Association
Fig. 9.4.2 Copyright 2003 Steve Dakin, reproduced with permission
Fig. 9.5 From Galton, F. (1910). Numeralised profiles for classification and recognition. *Nature, 83*, 127-130 with permission of Nature Publishing
Fig. 9.6 Copyright 2003 Michael Morgan
Fig. 9.7 Copyright 2003 Michael Morgan
Fig. 9.8 From http://www-white.media.mit.edu/vismod/demos/facerec/basic.html with permission of MIT Media Lab. The average face at top left is not the same as the original reason for technical reasons and is based on the average face from the Web site http://www.octapod.org.au/webdweller/averageface/ as of 19/08/2003
Fig. 9.9 From Leopold, D., O'Toole, A., T, & Blanz, V. (2001). Prototype-references shape encoding revealed by high-level aftereffects. *Nature Neuroscience, 4*, 89-94 with permission of the authors and Nature Publishing
Fig. 10.1 Copyright 2003 Michael Morgan
Fig. 10.2 Copyright 2003 Michael Morgan
Fig. 10.3 From Figure 1 (p 202) in Driver, J & Vuilleumier, P "Neglect' in the Encyclopedia of Cognitive Science, edited by Lynn Nadel with permission of the authors and Macmillan
Fig. 11.1 Reprinted with permisssion from Batista, A., Burneo, C., Snyder, L., & Andersen, R. A. (1999). Reach plans in eye-centered coordinates. *Science, 285*, 257-241. Copyright 1999 American Association for the Advancement of Science
Fig. 12.1 Copyright 2003 Steve Dakin, reproduced with permission
Fig. 15.1 Fig 85 from K. Brodmann (1909) Vergleichende Localisationslehre der Grosshirnrinde. Leipzig: Barth
Fig. 15.2 Copyright 2003 Josh Solomon, reproduced with permission
Fig. 16.1 From Cavanagh, P. (2002) Seeing the forest but not the trees, Nature Neuroscience, 4, 673 with permission of the authors and Nature Publishing
Fig. 16.2 From Milner, A., & Gooddale, M. (1995). The Visual Brain in Action. *Oxford: Oxford University Press* (Fig. 5.2, p. 128) with permission of the authors and Oxford University Press, and Nature Publishing (Vol 349, p 154)

PLATE SECTION

Plate (Thatcher Illusion). Copyright 2002 by Peter Thompson, reproduced with permission
Plate Section (Pinwheel Map). From Hubener, M., Shoham, D., Grinvald, A., & Bonhoeffer, T. (1997). Spatial relationships among three columnar systems in cat area 17. *Journal of Neuroscience, 17(23)*, 9270-9284. Copyright by the

Society for Neuroscience, reproduced with permission of the Society and the authors.

Plate (Multiple visual areas). Adapted from Van Essen, D.C (2003) Organization of visual areas in Macaque and human cerebral cortex. In : The Visual Neurosciences, L. Chalupa and J.S Werner, eds MIT Press (in press) with permission of the author.

Plate Section (Les Cinq Sens). Musée de l'Oeuvre de Notre Dame, Strasbourg (Bridgeman Art Library).

Plate Section (Poverty Map). Copyright British Library of Political and Economic Science, reproduced with permission

Plate Section 5 (Signorelli). Pinacoteca di Brera, Milan (Bridgeman Art Library).

Plate Section (reverse phi). Copyright George Mather 2003, reproduced with permission

Plate Section 8 (Bill Phillips water computer). Science & Society Picture Library, reproduced with permission.

Plate Section (La Poudreuse). Courtauld Institute Gallery, Somerset House, London (Bridgeman Art Library).

Plate ('Non' from *Guardian*). Popperfoto.com (Reuters/Yves Herman).

Plate (Las Meninas). Prado, Madrid (Bridgeman Art Library).

Plate (Death of Marat). Musées Royaux des Beaux-Arts de Belgique, Brussels (Bridgeman Art Library).

Plate (Treisman). Reprinted with permission of the authors from Fig. 23.32 in Howard, I. P., & Rogers , B. J. (2002). Seeing in depth., *Toronto: I. Porteous.* , adapted from A. Treisman (1962) Binocular rivalry and stereoscopic depth perception, Quarterly J. Exp. Psychol.,14,23-37.

Plate (Diaz-Canaja). From Fig. 2 in Alais, D., O'Shea, R., Mesana-Alais, C., & Wilson, I. (2000). On binocular alternation. *Perception, 29,* 1137-1445, with permission of the authors and Pion Publishing.

Preface

'The Mazy Course'

The prize for the worst poem about science has yet to be awarded. A possible winner is Cowley's poetic preface to Thomas Sprat's *History of the Royal Society*, nominated by Erich Heller as 'the first significantly ludicrous poem ever written'. The poem praises Chancellor Bacon for his support of Science, an 'injur'd Pupil' (male) who has been cruelly force-fed by philosophers with 'Desserts of Poetry' and, believe it or not, with 'wanton Wit':

> Bacon at last, a mighty Man arose,
> Whom a wise King and Nature chose
> Lord Chancellor of both their Laws,
> And boldly undertook the injur'd Pupil's cause.

The zoological lines of John Hookham Frere in 1799 have also received a mention:

> The feather'd race with pinions skims the air
> Not so the mackerel and still less the bear.

This is stiff competition, but my own favourite is by the respectable banker Samuel Rogers (1763–1855), whose laureateship, according to Chambers, was 'a tribute rather to his age than to his verse':

> Lulled in the countless chambers of the brain
> Our thoughts are link'd by many a hidden chain;
> Awake but one, and lo! what myriads arise!
> Each stamps its image as the other flies;

> Each thrills the seat of sense, that sacred source,
> Whence the fine nerves direct their mazy course.

Rogers' meandering picture of the brain has not worn well and the idea of a single 'seat of sense' is dead. Or is it? An old idea beginning to resurface is that 'consciousness' will be discovered in some specific part of the brain – perhaps the frontal lobes. The search for this 'seat of sense' has been compared to the quest for the Holy Grail. To the modern seeker after the Holy Grail, consciousness is, it seems, like a carburettor or coil, rather than being distributed like oil in an engine. The search for the elusive seat of consciousness is rather a large topic – too large, one might suspect, to allow a simple scientific solution, and doomed eventually to disappear, like the question 'What is Life?' There have been too many recent books on consciousness, and this one will not add further to their mazy course. Instead, it will focus on a more specific problem.

How do we see the space outside our bodies? We see a three-dimensional world in which objects such as trees and other people have definite locations, both with respect to one another and to ourselves. I take for granted what Francis Crick calls the 'astonishing hypothesis' that all our experience depends upon events in our brain – in other words, that science will one day provide a full and complete explanation of the contents of our consciousness. But what kinds of activities in the brain could be responsible for our visual perception of space? Philosophers and neuroscientists talk about the brain containing 'representations' of the outside world – appearances under another form, or 're-presentations'. Familiar examples of representations in everyday life are mirror images, paintings and maps. A map represents spatial information in a condensed form. But is this the right way to think about representation of space in the brain? We don't expect to find colours or smells in the brain, so why should we expect to find maps there?

I take a cartographer's view. Maps do exist in the brain, and they are the basis for our perception of space. I side with philosophers like Berkeley and Lotze who argue that the key to understanding our experience of space is that we have to move our bodies about in it; and to do this we need maps. When we are seeing, the eye receives rays from different directions in physical space; the brain then has to produce actions located in the physical space from which that light originates. The earliest stage of vision involves an image in the eye, followed by a crude map at the back of the head. I think it is becoming clear that as neuroscientists follow the connection between these maps and action, they will find a succession of maps, in which the spatial element is always present and vital for the next stage. There will be no mysterious sidings on this track from vision to action at which the map disappears to be replaced by 'visual awareness of space'. The visual awareness of space quite simply is identical to the activity in the maps leading from the retina to action. I do not believe that a mysterious entity called 'consciousness' will be found in one of these maps alone; the state of consciousness at any one time is the state of the whole pathway from vision to action, perhaps not even excluding the retina. The idea that activity in the eyes might contribute something to consciousness is distinctly unfashionable, to say the least. Examination of this heresy will require a logical analysis of what it might mean to 'localise' consciousness anywhere, and a critical examination of recent techniques like functional brain imagining, which are touted as searching for the 'Holy Grail' of consciousness in the brain. I argue that the search for this particular Holy Grail will be any more successful than the original.

Every day, the story runs, a man left the factory in which he worked carrying his tools in a wheelbarrow. The security guards had a tip-off that he was stealing from the factory, and every day they carefully checked his wheelbarrow; but they found only his tools. He was, of course, stealing wheelbarrows. Every day, another story runs, a neuroscientist patiently traced the signal from the retina of the eye, through the brain and eventually back to the muscles that move the eyes and the rest of the body. He wanted to find out where Space was represented. He found orderly maps of the image on the retina; he found maps that transformed the retinal map into 'pre-motor' maps and into 'motor' maps. Eventually he understood every step in the pathway leading from the retina to action, but he never found the consciousness of Space. He gave up, a disappointed man, making the same mistake as the guards who ignored the wheelbarrows.

The idea that the brain contains maps is old, and is often said to be uninteresting. It might have something to do with the mere mechanics of brain development, or with some equally boring constraints; but it sheds no light on our experience. According to this view, the real problem is not to find more and more maps in the brain, but to find how space is represented in a symbolic, non-spatial form; otherwise we are just begging the question. This view dates back to the theory of the early Christian philosophers that the soul has no spatial extension, and to the debate about 'angels on pinheads': but why should we follow this venerable opinion? It is perverse to try to eliminate space from the visual map in the brain, only to resuscitate it again to explain action in space.

An alternative, which puts maps back centre stage, is that the brain is a kind of analogue computer. An analogue computer represents the world as an internal space-time model that obeys the laws of physics. It differs from a digital computer that represents the world as numbers. Analogue computers are machines that do not have to translate their inputs into numbers before doing computations. The components of the brain – the nerve cells – are certainly analogue computers in this sense. They add, subtract, divide and multiply electrical signals arriving along their input lines. Special 'motion-detecting' cells in the brain are sophisticated analogue computers for calculating 'spatio-temporal energy'; other cells compare the image in the two eyes using a similar analogue computation. We shall meet many other examples, based on the ubiquitous analogue computer called the 'receptive field'. Neuroscientists need no persuading that the brain is a rich collection of analogue computers. However, many philosophers of artificial intelligence (AI) argue that the distinction between analogue and digital computing is irrelevant. They say that any operation of any analogue computer can be simulated by a PC. This is true; but simulation merely tells us that the operation of the analogue machine can be described by equations. The goal of theoretical neuroscience is to describe the operations of the brain by mathematical equations, and in this sense a digital computer might be able to simulate some aspects of brain functioning. This does not mean that the contents of our consciousness are identical to those equations. You don't need to be a weatherman to know that there is a difference between simulation of the global weather pattern on a computer and how the real wind blows. Computer programs do not cause tempests.

One of the most useful comments I have seen on theories of consciousness was on a T-shirt at a neuroscience conference. Under a picture of a brain, the legend read: 'I think the brain is the most important and complicated organ in the body. But *Hey, who's telling me this?*' A good question indeed, when you are puzzled by the theory that there would be no consciousness without language, or that consciousness resides in an 'executive controller', who keeps the unruly parts of the brain in order. Perhaps these messages are coming from the language faculty, or from the aspiring executive controller himself. For obvious reasons, we should be particularly suspicious of claims coming from the language centres of the brain, which have a virtual monopoly on communication in our verbose society. Maybe when the language nerve cells tell us that they are responsible for consciousness they should be told to get out more, to a football match or to the ballet. When Dr Johnson was asked to refute Berkeley's denial of the existence of matter, he did not waste time on language: he kicked the stone instead.

Theories of consciousness are divided by one Great Schism, and several minor ones. The Great Schism is between those who think that consciousness will be understood from the anatomy and physiology of the brain, and those who think that it will be understood by writing computer programs to simulate it. According to the first view, the nature of our sensations is completely determined by the structure of our brains. Other machines may or may not have awareness, but there is no reason to think that it has anything in common with *our* awareness: the states of mind of a non-brain are literally unimaginable. According to the second view – strong AI, as it is called – computers programmed to simulate the workings of the brain will have exactly the same experiences as ourselves.

Neuroscientists, for obvious reasons, tend to favour the first view; but it is a notoriously difficult theory to sell to our brains. If different conscious states correspond to the activity of different conglomerations of cells in the brain, what is it about these cells that explains the different experiences? Most brains seem to feel that there is some ineffable gap to be crossed between the activity of brain cells and our conscious awareness. Even with 'simple' sensations such as that of colour, how can the firing of some nerve cells make us see 'red' and the firing of other cells make us experience 'blue'? Can we, in fact, ever hope to identify sensations with particular nerve cells in the brain? Millions of words have been written on this problem of 'qualia' – as it is called – without solving it. Hard though it may be to accept, the problem appears to be one that our ordinary language is incapable of solving, rather like the problems addressed by quantum theory. This book will not attempt to solve the problem. Instead, it will concentrate on the much more modest goal of analysing what sort of experimental evidence we would need to tie down our awareness of the outside world to a particular part of the brain. An especially intriguing possibility is that many parts of the brain, even of the cerebral cortex, are unconscious automata, with no more awareness than the autopilot in an aircraft. If this is so, how would we know it to be true?

The book as a whole is divided into four parts. The first deals with the nature of images, and the differences between images and maps. It starts with Bishop Berkeley's argument that seeing is not the same as having an image, and ends with the problem of how we see the third dimension. On the way it describes how maps are formed during development of the brain, how frogs can use maps for simple tasks such as catching flies and how the two eyes combine in the human brain.

The second part is about analogue computers and the nature of analogue computations in the brain. It introduces the idea that the brain generates its own perceptions in the form of internal models, which it checks for accuracy against incoming sensory data. Analogue computations in the brain are illustrated by the perception of movement and our ability to recognise complex objects such as individual human faces.

The third part is about the way our body influences the perception of space and includes an account of the puzzling 'neglect' syndrome in which patients apparently ignore the left side of space even though they are not blind to it.

The fourth and final part asks whether we have any reason to put conscious awareness in one part of the brain rather than another. It begins with the evidence that we see much less than we think we do and analyses the idea that large areas of the brain make no contribution to awareness. It criticises the idea that nerve cells secrete sensations 'as the liver secretes bile' – an idea often discussed and dismissed as a straw man, but close to recent claims that some nerve cells make a 'direct' contribution to conscious awareness.

I have tried to avoid technical terms and jargon, such as 'neurones' for 'nerve cells'. An exception is the shorthand word 'observer' to describe the person taking part in an experiment or looking at any image. Being British makes me averse to the alternative term 'subject'. The word 'observer' has a long and honourable history in astronomy and aviation. 'Movie' is used instead of 'film' or the cumbersome 'motion picture'. It is accepted by the OED. The book is not written for (or about) scientists, but if any scientists do venture inside, they may find the following translations helpful:

Nerve cell – *neuron(e)*
Nerve fibre – *axon*
Front – *anterior*
Back – *posterior*
Top – *dorsal*
Bottom – *ventral*
Hallucinating faces with prominent teeth – *Prosopometamorphosia*
Exaggerated attention to shiny objects – *Hyperprosessis*

Many thanks to colleagues who have read the text in whole or in part and corrected my errors; those that remain are my responsibility alone. I owe an especial debt to Mitch Glickstein for communicating to me his wonderul enthusiasm for neuroscience. I hope he writes his own book one day; it will be better than mine. Linda Partridge not only read the book and made many helpful suggestions from the standpoint of a geneticist, but put up with me when I was writing it. To my long-suffering research colleagues: I promise to get back to the bench next week.

PART ONE
IMAGES AND MAPS

1

Murder on the Highway

Type the words 'retina', 'murder' and 'image' into a Web search engine and one is soon led to the novel 'The Story of Sevenoaks', written in 1875 by the popular Dr J. G. Holland. 'Sevenoaks' has not worn well, but here is a résumé: 'General' Belcher, President of the Crooked Valley Railroad, and purveyor of the suspect Belcher rifle to the Prussian government, has forged the signature of Nicholas Johnston, for personal advantage. He is confronted in court by an expert on handwriting and chemistry. The expert is certain that the disputed signature is a forgery. It is too perfect to be other than a tracing; moreover, under magnification it is seen to have the slight unsteadiness characteristic of tracing. Professor Tims offers to show the enlarged signature to the jury with the help of a solar lanthorn. This sets the stage for the melodramatic chapter *'In which a Heavenly Witness Appears Who Cannot be Cross-Examined, and before which the Defence Breaks down utterly'*. The source of light for the projector is the Sun – the 'Heavenly Witness ... Who Cannot be Cross-Examined'. The astonished silence following projection of the signature is broken by the hollow groan, *'Mene, mene, tekel upharsin!'* 'Balshazzar, on his night of doom, could hardly have presented a more pitiful front than Robert Belcher, when all eyes were turned on him.'

But should a photographic image be admissible as evidence in a court of law? This was a matter of dispute just after the development of photography, just as the validity of DNA evidence is disputed today. Any new scientific technique will be challenged by defence lawyers trying to discredit evidence that might put their client in jail. No sooner did photographs appear in court than forensically inspired doubt was thrown on the accuracy of lenses. The 'witness who could not be cross-examined' is neatly confounded by the dismissing of photographs as 'hearsay of the sun'. To these objections, however, there was a crushing scientific rejoinder:

> Science has discovered that a perfect photograph of an object, reflected in the eye of one dying, remains fixed in the retina after death. (See recent experiments stated by Dr. Vogel in the May number 1877 of Philadelphia Photographic Journal). Take the case of a murder committed on the highway; on the eye of the victim is fixed the perfect likeness of a human face. Would the court exclude the knowledge of that fact from the jury, on the trial of the man against whom the glazed eye of the murdered man thus bore testimony?

In other words, if our vision itself depends on a photographic image in the retina, there can be no valid objection to using other forms of photographs as evidence. The belief that a dead person might have a retinal imprint of his murderer on his retina was widespread in the nineteenth century and apparently survived in Dublin up to 16 June 1904 (Bloomsday), since its appearance in a newspaper article is referred to in *Ulysses* (*'Murder. The murderer's image in the eye of the murdered. They love reading about it.'*). The first 'Optogram' was made by 1876 by Willy Kühne, Professor of Physiology at the University of Heidelberg, who managed to form a faint image of a barred window in the eye of an albino rabbit. Optograms are formed because the visual pigment (stored in special cells, called rods and cones, in the retina) loses its deep red colour when exposed to light. The great German physicist Helmholtz was delighted when Kühne sent him news of the optogram: 'I have been immensely pleased with this find; I had always imagined hypothetically that there must be some photo-chemical action in the retina, but had never supposed one would be able to demonstrate it.' We now know that Helmholtz was right: the energy of light is trapped by special pigments in rods and cones. When these pigments – called 'opsins' – absorb light, they set in train a long series of chemical reactions within the rods and cones, culminating in the sending of an electrical message along the optic nerve to the brain. There are many different opsins in nature, each one responding best to a particular wavelength of light. The human brain compares the output of three different opsins (in three different kinds of cone) to give us our colour vision.

The 'recent experiments stated by Dr. Vogel in the May number 1877 of Philadelphia Photographic Journal' are merely a description of Kühne's experiments. For reasons that remain inscrutable, Dr Vogel begins by proclaiming that he has come not to advertise a new hair oil in the manner of a 'Parisian Friseur'. He is, however, able to inform the reader that 'the natural laws of sight are discovered'. Dr Vogel predicts that the discovery of 'sight purple' will lead to other discoveries of substances sensitive to light, which may be of great advantage to photography. He bases this opinion on the 'astonishing sensitiveness' of our sight, which 'can distinguish very easily all details in the darkest corner of the room in a moment, while in photography it takes an exposure of hours to receive a poor picture'. Here Dr Vogel was misled. Progress in photography did not depend on copying the eye, and the wonders of vision are not to be found in the sensitivity of visual purple, but in the brain.

Optograms made a deep impression on the public imagination, but do not support the idea that an image will be fixed on the eye at the instant of death. A convent school in Liverpool taught me that the soul must differ from the body because there is no chemical difference between the body in the instants before and after death. Like other pieces of information from the same source, this has turned out to be not entirely accurate. The chemical reactions in the brain and eye change as soon as we die, including the absorption of light by the visual pigments. Unless the murderer's image were fixed in alum (as Kühne fixed his rabbit's eye), it would be soon disappear. The disappointment of Scotland Yard when they failed in 1888 to find Jack the Ripper's picture in the eye of his victim Annie Chapman was scientifically predictable.

The eye does indeed form an image on the retina, but its purpose is not as obvious as that of an image in a camera. Like TV and movie images, the picture taken by a camera is ultimately destined to be shown to the human eye, and thus to form a retinal image. The retinal image itself, however has not been designed to be looked at by the human eye; and this is fortunate, because the retinal image is very imperfect compared to the images of cameras and telescopes. Take the perception of 'blur', for example. We are normally quite unaware that the image on the retina is always somewhat blurred, owing to imperfections in the optics of the eye. We see an image as perfectly sharp when it is as well focused as the imperfect eye can make it, not when it is perfectly focused. This makes sense if we think of perceived blur not as some ghostly internal equivalent of optical blur, but instead as an invitation to focus the eye. The brain learns to tolerate a certain amount of optical blur in the image and considers it as normal. Indeed,

Blur adapt   Sharp adapt

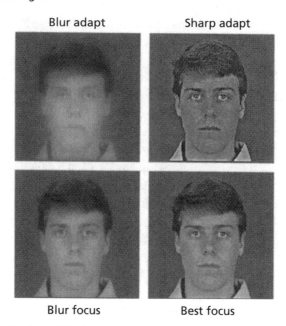

Blur focus   Best focus

Figure 1.1 Adapting to blur (top) changes the perception of best focus (bottom)

the amount of blur that the brain considers 'normal' can be changed by looking at blurred photographs. After staring for a few minutes at the blurred photograph of a face, observers think that slightly blurred photographs are preferable to normal ones (see figure 1.1), proof that even an optical image quality such as blur is actively interpreted by the brain, rather than being merely copied.

The problem that has dogged the philosophy of visual perception is that seeing begins with an image – the optical image in the retina – and ends in a completely different kind of image – our perceptual image of the world outside. Because we use the same term – 'image' – for both kinds (in European languages, at any rate), we are tempted to confuse the properties of the two kinds of image. Healthy mental exercises are needed to cure ourselves of this bad habit. So take a deep breath, and begin by asking the apparently bizarre question: why do we bother to make an image on the retina at all? Plants, fungi and bacteria don't bother. Some molluscs do, but cannot perceive shapes. Flies have hundreds of images. We have two. Why this diversity?

The message from the evolution of the eye is that 'big is beautiful'. Unlike most organs, the eye does not increase in proportion to body size, because its optical performance depends on its absolute, not its relative size. The sparrow's eye is as large as its brain and all its other sense organs put together. Even so, it is no match for the eyes of larger animals. The ostrich has the record for land-living animals, with an eye 50mm in diameter, which enables it to see a bump on the ground 2m high at a distance of 24km. Horses, zebras and other plain-dwelling animals are not far behind: their bulging eyes are early-warning systems, designed to detect approaching danger over large distances. Whales have eyes as large as footballs. Birds of prey such as hawks and eagles have exceptionally large eyes, which they use for spotting prey from the air. If they could be tested with an eye chart, they would read one more line than ourselves.

A good reason for having a large eye is that large eyes gather more light. Light enters the eye through the pupil, and the area of the pupil determines how much light it lets through. The larger the telescope the fainter the stars it can see, and it is the same with the eye; but this only works if the image is focused. If the image is unfocused, the rays of light from an object spread all over the retina, and since the area of the retina is exactly proportional to the area of the pupil, we should gain nothing from making the eye larger. However, if the image is focused, all the rays of light from a distant point of light are brought together at the same point on the retina (which is, after all, what 'focus' means) and they stimulate the same rod or cone. The rods and cones work more reliably and more quickly when they get more light, so here we have an excellent reason both for the larger eye, and for a focusing mechanism within it.

If gathering as much light as possible were the only problem the eye had to solve, the pupil would always be as large as possible; but this is only part of the story: as we all know, the pupil decreases its size in bright light. Part of the reason may be to protect the retina from getting too much illumination – like too much oxygen, too much light is toxic and it kills rods and cones; but there is another reason, arising from the defective nature of the eye as an optical instrument. The eye has historically been in the front rank of organs held to prove the skill of the Creator and the impossibility of producing such a complex machine by blind chance; yet the inventor of the ophthalmoscope, Hermann von Helmholtz, said that God should have been ashamed of such a shoddy instrument as the human eye. The main problems are the cornea and the lens, which are not quite the right shape to focus all the rays of light on to the same point of the retina. Rays going through the edges of the lens are brought to a different point from those going through the centre. The only way the eye can prevent this is by closing down the pupil to exclude these marginal rays.

This becomes cruelly obvious with advancing age, and deterioration of vision is usually our first intimation of mortality. Deterioration of the eye begins, like the decline of sexual potency, at the age of fifteen, but the ageing lens, unlike the ageing penis, becomes stiff and hard. Reading becomes difficult without glasses, and particularly so when trying to read in dim light. In dim light the pupil expands to pump more light into the eye, but in doing so it defocuses the image, preventing reading. If there is enough light, visual acuity can be improved with a 'pinhole' pupil. Pinholes were the earliest kind of reading aid and they are still on the market today. Punch a hole in a piece of paper with a needle and look through the hole at a brightly lit page of text; it is possible to read from a distance as small as one inch from the page. The trick does not work under dim light, because the pinhole does not let through enough light to see by. A bizarre attempt to get round this involves opaque glasses punched with hundreds of pinholes, which are collectively supposed to supply enough light. However, looking like an insect is rather a high price to pay for clear vision.

Age is only one cause of problems with the retinal image. The male children of Orthodox Jews in the London district of Stamford Hill have something in common with many Japanese, and with a group of children in an infamous study of IQ carried out in California in the 1930s. Large numbers of the ultra-Orthodox Jewish boys – but not their sisters – are reported anecdotally to be myopic: they can read very small print at close distances, but cannot see distant objects so well. When I taught a graduate class in Japan, every single student wore lenses for far vision. The myopic Californians had higher IQs than their less owlish contemporaries. The common link may be close reading, whether it be the tiny characters in the commentaries to the Talmud, the very subtle differences between Kanji ideograms, or the books in the homes of wealthier Californians (IQ being, if nothing else, a reliable measure of parental income). If the eye is used mainly for close work, perhaps it becomes adapted to focus on nearby objects rather than ones in the distance, and myopia results.

There is nothing inherently defective about the moderately myopic eye: it is simply adapted to a different viewing distance from the so-called 'normal' eye; but how does it get that way? The eye is not a finished product at birth: it has to grow from 17 mm at birth to its adult size of 24 mm, and a difference of only a few tenths of a millimetre can make the difference between the normal and myopic eye. The myopic eye is too long for the focusing power of its lens and cornea, with the result that the image of a distant object is focused in front of the retina. One theory of how the eye gets to be the 'correct' size is that it keeps growing until the nerve cells in the retina signal that the image is in focus. If chickens are reared with a spectacle lens in front of one eye, that eye compensates to some extent by growing to a different size from that of the normal chick. The correction does not cross over to the other eye, and does not depend on a connection of the eye to the brain. Perhaps some eyes become myopic because they are given a diet of too much close work during development; but there is no proof of this in people as yet.

The original purpose of forming an image in the eye may have been to increase the amount of light falling on the photoreceptors, but there are obvious additional benefits. In a focused image, light rays coming from different directions in space end up at different points on the retina and give information about the location of objects in space. The advantages of having an image may seem obvious, but merely having an image is not enough. The point of an image is not to have it, but to interpret it. To use the image, our brain has to carry out measurements on the image, the first of which is to compare the number of photons absorbed by different rods and cones. A hovering kestrel is exquisitely sensitive to the slightest movement of its prey and can detect movement from changes of as little as 2 per cent in the amount of light falling on a cone. The sharper and more magnified the image, the smaller the movement of the prey that will correspond to this 2 per cent difference. Several birds of prey have hit on the trick of finding small rodents by locating their droppings, which glow strongly at the ultraviolet end of the spectrum. To do this, they have to measure very small differences in UV between neighbouring photoreceptors in the image. The better focused and more magnified the image, the more sensitive this and other kinds of contrast detection will be.

One of the first philosophers to say that we have to interpret the retinal image was George Berkeley (1685–1753), who published his 'Essay towards a New Theory of Vision' when he was only twenty-four years old. Berkeley is infamous for his much parodied denial of the existence of matter:

> There was once a man who said, 'God
> Must think it exceedingly odd

> If he finds that this tree
> Continues to be
> When there's no one about in the Quad.'

And the reply:

> 'Dear Sir, your astonishment's odd:
> I am always about in the Quad.
> And that's why the tree
> Will continue to be,
> Since observed by Yours Faithfully, God.'

Berkeley's philosophy eventually led him to deny altogether the existence of matter and a world outside the mind. His theory has not proved popular. 'I refute it *thus*,' said Dr Johnson, by striking his foot against a large stone until it rebounded. But the scepticism that led Berkeley in the end to his philosophical idealism began innocently enough, with some questions about the retinal image.

The main point of the 'New Theory' is to show that the properties of the retinal image are very different from our visual perceptions – so different, indeed, that visual perception is not an optical image at all: what we call vision is actually a memory of the past, derived in the first place from touch and movement. Berkeley begins his attack on the retinal image with a bang, right in the second paragraph of the 'Essay', by pointing out that rays of light arriving at the eye give no information about the distance they have travelled: 'It is, I think, agreed by all that distance, of itself and immediately, cannot be seen. For distance being a Line directed end-wise to the eye, it projects only one point in the fund of the eye, which remains invariably the same, whether the distance be longer or shorter.'

This is perfectly true: distance is not given directly in the image. Indeed, we can see distance in images that are really flat, the obvious examples being photographs and paintings. Moreover, the perception of the size of objects is just as much a problem. The image of a man shrinks in size as he walks away, yet we do not perceive him as becoming a dwarf. And if anyone should still think that our perceptions are copies of the retinal image, says Berkeley, they should consider the fact that the retinal image is upside down. 'Since therefore the pictures are thus inverted, it is demanded how it comes to pass that we see the objects erect and in their natural position.'

Berkeley's solution was to say that experience comes to our aid and teaches us to associate visual impressions with the true properties of objects. By moving about the world we learn that further objects are partly hidden behind nearer ones, and that their images are smaller and fainter. This is what makes the Moon on the horizon seem larger than the Moon high in the sky. We no more *see* the true size and distance of objects, says Berkeley, than we *see* anger and shame in the looks of a man. We *infer* size and distance just as we infer the existence of invisible passions, by association of ideas. Visual sensations have no resemblance to the properties of objects. They are entirely arbitrary symbols like the words in a language, which could have had a quite different meaning, or like the signs that put red lines through symbols (see figure 1.2). In Berkeley's strange world, the image of a tall building could suggest to us a doll's house, and vice versa. 'Lesser visual magnitudes could have been associated with greater tangible magnitudes,' he says. If our eyes were microscopes, Berkeley comments, we should have no idea of how to interpret the images, and we would be left 'with only the empty amusement of seeing, without any other benefit arising from it.'

There is both good and bad news from modern neuroscience for Berkeley's theory of vision. He was right – and well ahead of his time – to question the naive conception of vision as a form of optical imagery. True, Descartes had earlier scorned the idea that the eye sends little images into the brain, but he gives the game away when he locates seeing in the tiny pineal gland, on the grounds that there is only one pineal. He wants to transform the image as much as possible into a mathematical point. Mental images for Descartes are immaterial and cannot have extension in space; therefore they are unlike optical

Figure 1.2 'Règlements' in Québec

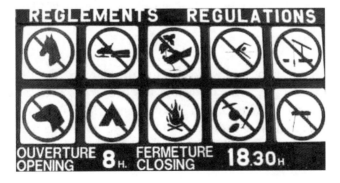

images. Like angels on pinheads, an infinite number of sensations could fit into the pineal gland. This is not the same reasoning as Berkeley's.

The bad news about the 'New Theory' is that it is wrong: the theory is not radical enough. Berkeley assumes that there are such things as visual sensations, and that these have properties such as size and position in space. In other words, Berkeley imagines a two-stage process of seeing, in the first of which we see the retinal image, and in the second, the tangible properties of objects; but this is to assume that we can somehow *directly* see the size of retinal images in the first place, and to ignore the logical point that some mechanism must exist, in the retina or in the brain, to measure the size of an image. Once we accept that size has to be measured, there is no need to suppose that the size of the retinal image appears first in consciousness, before the size of the object.

For example, the image of a tree on the retina is indeed upside down with respect to our body, but it would make no sense to have a two-stage process, first seeing the image upside down with respect to our body, and then the right way up. We see the top of a tree as higher than its roots because we have to move our eyes *upwards* to see the top clearly, says Berkeley; and once again, this is something we have to learn from our experience. But is it true that we have to learn to see the world the right way up? Berkeley was certainly not alone in thinking so. The need for 'experience' in interpreting our sensations is repeated like a mantra by all the philosophers of the Enlightenment, from Locke in England to the Abbé de Condillac in France. Here, for example, is Voltaire in the *Elements of Newton's Philosophy*, commenting on the perception of size:

> I see a great way off, through a little hole, a man upon the top of a house … As soon as I judge it to be a man, the connection implanted in my mind by experience between the idea of a man and the idea of a height from five to six feet, obliges me, without thinking of it, to imagine, by an instant judgement, that I see a man of such a height.

Just as endlessly repeated was the story of the man, blind from birth because of cataracts, who recovered the use of his eyes as an adult thanks to surgery. The Dublin lawyer James Molyneux asked John Locke whether such a patient would be able to distinguish by sight objects – such as a cube and a globe – which he had previously been able to distinguish by touch. Locke's answer was 'No': the man would have no names for his visual sensations until he learned to associate them with touch. The Abbé de Condillac had his own fable – that of the stone statue that emulates the Commander of Seville by coming to life and creaking off its pedestal; but unlike the Commander, Condillac's statue would have posed little menace to Don Juan, for he initially sees everything upside down. Only after experience does the lapidary incompetent finally see the light.'

It is no coincidence that the philosophers of the Enlightenment chose blindness as one of their main metaphors for fighting the ecclesiastical and civil authorities. The man born blind lacks the most important human sense; he has to rely on hearsay and the authority of others to know about the external world. He is in the position of people who rely upon the bishops and the philosophers of the ancient world for their ideas, rather than using the evidence of their own senses. Wake up and use your own senses, not the authority of others! The constant theme that we gain our knowledge only from experience is to be understood as a political statement, not merely as scientific speculation. Marx was wrong when he said, 'The Philosophers have only interpreted the world in various ways; the point is to change it.' John Locke's *Treatise of Civil Government* was as familiar as the Bible to the colonists of the American Revolution: the Enlightenment philosophers changed the Western world into a better place.

Some may therefore sympathise with the ideology behind Condillac's statue – but that does not make it a correct account of vision. The theory that our experience of visual space has to be learned in its entirety from touch and movement is wrong. Take the 'upside-down' retinal image as an example. Rays of light hitting the top half of the retina are seen as coming from the lower part of visual space, nearest to the ground; rays hitting the bottom half are seen as coming from the top half of space or sky. This can be experienced by exerting very gentle pressure on the eyelid (not the eye!). Pressure on the part of the top left eyelid nearest to the nose causes a spot to appear in the *lower* left part of the visual field: the effect is initially quite surprising because the spot and the point of pressure do not appear to 'line up'. Left and right are also reversed. Have we learned this association between position on the retina and direction is space, as Berkeley claimed? A beautiful experiment says not. In 1902 the German ophthalmologist Sclodtmann studied some blind patients who had been deprived of sight at or near the time of birth. When their eyeballs were pressed they saw points of light just like normal people and pointed to them as if they were coming from the same direction as that seen by normally sighted people. Therefore, the association between retinal position and direction in space is innate, not learned through experience. In a Nobel prize-winning experiment, the American neuroscientist Roger Sperry cut the optic nerve of a frog (which unlike ours will regenerate if cut) and replaced the eye upside down. The frog struck at flies as if the retinal image had been reversed up–down and left–right, proof that the nerves from, say, the top-left part of the eye grew back to the same part of the brain as they had connected to previously, and messages arriving from it were interpreted in exactly the same way. Learning cannot have been the explanation, for why would the frog learn to avoid catching its prey?

An explorer would soon learn that his map was reversed, and would adjust his navigation to suit. An inverting lens system or system of mirrors in front of the eye reverses the map on the retina. Do we learn to compensate? George Stratton tried this in an experiment that Richard Gregory has described as 'perhaps the most famous ... in the whole of experimental psychology'.

When Stratton first put on his inverting lenses, he saw the world upside down, and all his actions were reversed: reaching for a cup on a table in the lower part of their visual field, he would grasp at the air above his head, in the position where the cup was seen. He found it difficult to walk. By the sixth day, however, his performance had greatly improved, and he began (on his own account) to see the world the right way up. In a repeat of Stratton's experiment, volunteers wore upside-down inverting mirrors at Innsbruck University for up to two weeks during the years 1947–54; and with practice their movements quite rapidly improved. Within a few days they were able to ride a bicycle and even go skiing! The spectacular improvement of Kohler's volunteers seems to support Berkeley's contention that perception is a learned *interpretation* of the visual image. How, though, can we reconcile this with demonstration by pressing the eyeball that the perception of up and down is innate?

The tough question here is whether Stratton and Kohler had really learned to *see* the world 'the right way up', as opposed to coping with its appearing upside down. Given that they could ride a bicycle, the question may seem odd, but it makes sense. For example, squints can be treated by a prism that brings the images in the two eyes into register. The prism displaces the retinal image leftwards or rightwards, depending on its rotation relative to the eye. If a normally sighted observer puts prisms in front of *both eyes* (so that the images in both eyes are displaced to the right), they are disoriented and grasp empty air to the *left* of an object they are trying to pick up; but they adapt within a few minutes and reach for objects correctly. Have they learned to see the objects in the right position relative to their bodies? No, for if they learn to reach correctly with their left arm, they have to learn all over again when tested with their right arm. Their new talent is a trick with one of their arms, not a genuine shift in perception of the object relative to the *whole* body. The same observer points in the wrong direction when trying to locate a sound coming from an invisible loudspeaker. They have adjusted the position of their arm in their map of outside space, not their perception of the position of objects in space.

The right-hand image of a famous face in figure 1.3 looks grotesque because the mouth and eyes have been pasted upside down. Turning the page upside down makes the face look reasonably normal. We can infer from this that our perception of the expression in the mouth and eyes depends in part on whether they are right way up or wrong way up relative to the *retina*, rather than relative to the nose and rest of the face. How would this image look after adapting for a period of days to an inverting mirror? If we think that experience with inverting mirrors teaches us to invert the image on the retina, a simple prediction suggests itself. At first, when we put the inverting mirrors on, the image should look upside down and benign, but after adaptation it should look the right way up – and grotesque. In other words, it should look just like it

Figure 1.3 Thompson's Thatcher illusion

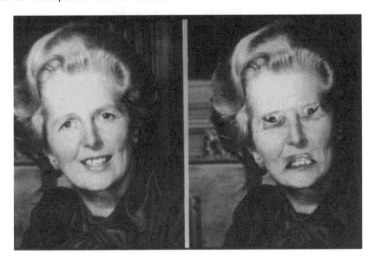

does to us in our unadapted state when we turn the page upside down. The alternative, if no genuine rotation has taken place, is that the face will still seem to smile.

This experiment has not been done, but a similar one has. The image in figure 1.4 shows shaded discs. On the left, all but one look like bumps coming out of the page; the 'odd man out' looks like a crater. The explanation is that we have specialised neural circuits for determining 'shape from shading', and these work on the assumption that light comes from the top of the image, as it usually does in nature. If the page is turned upside down the bumps become hollows and vice versa. Observers with inverting lenses also see the bumps and hollows reversed, as we should expect. If, after adaptation, they had somehow turned the image around inside their heads, they should eventually overcome the reversal of bumps and hollows. In the experiment, none of the observers switched bumps into craters after adaptation. The powers of learning are severely limited.

Reading tells the same story. All observers in the bumps and craters experiment learned to read inverted script. This is not surprising, for we can all learn to read upside-down or mirror-imaged script given a bit of practice. Leonardo da Vinci and many others have perfected the art of mirror writing, but none of the observers has said that they learned to see the script the right way up during the experiment.

We now come to the heart of the matter: how can observers see objects the wrong way up but still ride bicycles? The facts make no sense if we think that perception is an internal image. Our brains use the image on the retina for many different purposes. One is to guide our movements, and the inverting mirror experiments seem to show that this system can learn rapidly when the retinal image is inverted. The other sees the shape of objects and their orientation with respect to gravity and is much less flexible than the first when the image is

Figure 1.4 Bumps and hollows

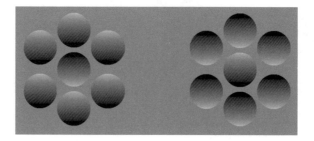

inverted. We cannot learn to see an upside-down face as normal, or at least not easily; but we can learn rapidly to point correctly at its mouth. We shall see later that the division between these two systems may correspond with two different anatomical circuits in the brain, one flowing towards the control of movement; the other towards the recognition of faces and other shapes. The message from neuroscience is that there is no single internal image of 'space' in the brain. However, this does not mean that there are no maps at all: on the contrary, the brain takes its maps very seriously, as the next chapter will show.

2

Conventional Signs

The Emperor Napoleon invaded Russia in June 1812 with an army half a million strong. In December of the same year La Grande Armée struggled back across the Berezina river with only 10,000 men. Even these might not have survived without the leadership of Marshal Michel Ney, himself practically the last member of the army to leave Russia (on 14 December). Napoleon had already abandoned the remnants of the army on 5 December. The disastrous fate of the army is chronicled in a famous map (1861) by Charles Joseph Minard, a retired inspector of France's equivalent of the Department of Transport. Minard's map (see figure 2.1) shows the main rivers and towns on Napoleon's march and two bands, one indicating the route to Moscow and the other the route back. The width of each band is proportional to the size of the army. We can also read the rapidly falling temperature (in degrees Réaumur) from a scale on the bottom of the map.

This chapter is about maps in the brain, and their differences from images. An image is simply a pattern of light and dark on a surface; a map is a tool for conveying information. The most obvious purpose of a map is to give us information about distance and direction. A map usually has a scale from which distances can be read and a direction with respect to a known standard. However, there are many functions a map can serve even if it fails to convey distances. The well-known 1931 London Underground map by Harry Beck, drawn according to the conventions of an electrical wiring diagram, tells us how the stations are connected, but not how far they are apart above ground.

Nor are maps confined to representing space. Minard's map represents not only space but time. Colour is often pressed into service in maps as an additional source of information. In Charles Booth's 1899 'poverty map' of London, colour represents income (see plate section).

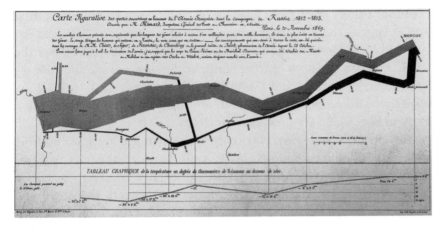

Figure 2.1 Minard's map of Napoleon's 1812–13 Russian campaign

Wyld's 1815 'Chart of Civilisations' colours countries from 'I' (very uncivilised) to 'V' (England). Canada gets an unkind II for containing 'cannibals and Frenchmen': it is not clear whether it was the cannibals or the French who raised it above Australia (I).

Contrast this use of colour with a simple image. The yellowness of a banana in a photograph is not put there as a symbol of a banana. Sometimes the difference between a symbol and an image is easily lost, as when looking at a pseudo-coloured image from the Hubble telescope. Is that star coloured blue because it sends out short wavelength light, or to symbolise the fact that it has only just been born? The ambiguity between symbol and image delighted surrealist painters such as Magritte.

Unlike a map, a photograph contains a large amount of information but in a completely undigested form. We cannot read directions or distances from an image, because there is no scale or compass. It is meaningless to say that one point is to the north of another in the image on the retina, or that two points are from objects a nautical mile apart. An image is just an image – a splattering of light on a two-dimensional surface. Magritte's famous image of a pipe is entitled '*Ceci n'est pas une pipe*'. He means (I think): it's an image.

In Lewis Carroll's 'The Hunting of the Snark' the Bellman tries to convert nautical maps into images. He derides 'Mercator's North Pole and Equators', and persuades the gullible crew that these are 'merely conventional signs'. He ends with an empty blue image. At the other extreme, a short story by Lewis Carroll describes a German map that was as large as the country it represented. 'It has never been spread out yet, said Mein Herr: the farmers objected; they said it would cover the whole country and shut out the sunlight! So now we use the country itself as its own map, and I assure you it does nearly as well.' (The uselessness of a map that is merely an image is also the theme of a story in Borges and Casares' *Extraordinary Tales*).

The distance between two points in an image tells us nothing about how long it would take us to walk between them. A nautical chart does. When we use a chart to work out a course to steer, we use an instrument like a Breton plotter to measure the angle and distance between the starting point and intended finishing point. But this makes sense only if we assume some numerical relationship between the map and the real world – a 'metric'. If the angle between two reasonably nearby points on the chart is 135 degrees, then you will get between them by steering south-east. If the distance between them is equal to two minutes of latitude on the vertical scale, it is two nautical miles – and so on. None of this would be possible on an image of the world taken from space. Even if you could identify Plymouth and the Eddystone Rock from the photograph, you would have no idea what course to steer between them, or how far they were apart.

The image on the retina is an image and nothing more. Where is it transformed into the maps we use to judge angles and distances, and to move around in our three-dimensional world? The first place where this could happen is in the retina itself. The retina is not a passive medium like a film in a camera, but a highly complicated outgrowth of brain itself. (It grows on the end of a stalk which pushes outwards from the brain during development.) The rods and cones are connected to several layers of interacting nerve cells, culminating in a layer that sends nerve fibres along the optic nerve. Suppose each nerve fibre in the optic nerve were to send out its own private call-sign, in the form of a pattern of nerve impulses that could be recognised by the brain: '*This is WCX Retina calling: here is the latest news about flying insects.*' A three-letter code could distinguish $26 \times 26 \times 26$, or 17,576, different retinal positions: good enough to catch flies. Of course, the retina cannot send out a code consisting of letters; but the unique signal or signature could, for example, be the precise time interval between successive nerve impulses sent along the nerve. The brain would then recognise the position of a spot of light on the retina just as it recognises a smell. Every smell has a unique quality, which depends on the pattern of activity in the different nerve fibres of the olfactory nerve. We can't easily describe the unique smell of a rose, but it has one. The first scientist to suggest that the retina generates unique signals like smells corresponding to positions was Herman Lotze, who called them 'local signs'.

Herman Lotze taught in Göttingen and his book *Medical Psychology* was published in 1852. Lotze was the first scientist to think deeply about how space might be represented in the nervous system. He rejects the naive idea that images are tranferred directly into the brain. British readers of a certain generation may remember 'The Numbskulls' in *Beezer*. The Numbskulls inhabit the cranium of their owner and do his thinking and perceiving for him. One Numbskull looks out through the eyes with a telescope and reports what he sees to other Numbskulls, who shout through megaphones to the mouth, and so on. Harmless stuff, but Lotze would have deplored the *Beezer* model of perception: 'Only a thoroughly childish way of thinking in earlier times spoke of pictures, which detached themselves from the outside world, and entered through the sense organs into the mind ... The mind is not a passive or extended medium in which spatial pictures of objects could occur.'

So much for childish theories, then; but if we abolish the egregious Numbskulls, what takes their place? Lotze would like to say that the spatial information in the image is retained in the brain as some form of map, but here he finds himself in difficulties. He has read Immanuel Kant and has convinced himself that maps in the brain cannot explain the perception of space. A simple summary of Kant's Philosophy of Perception explains why. Kant denied there could be any *direct* similarity between our perceptions of objects and objects 'in themselves'. The phrase 'in themselves' refers to properties the object would still have if there were no one to perceive it – 'no one about in the Quad', as the limerick about Berkeley has it. If cones had not evolved in the retina, the rainbow would have no colours. Fine, we might say, but there are some properties that objects really, *really* do have – such as the wavelength of the light they reflect. Not so, says Kant. Reflectance spectra and wavelengths of light are only ways in which we represent things to our mind. They are no more properties of 'things in themselves' than are colours. Space and Time themselves are mental representations of a world that is in itself unknowable. We cannot even call it the 'outside' world, because this would be to use a spatial representation. Kant has two rather different explanations of why we experience Space and Time. The first is that they are properties of our human cognition and ultimately of our brains. They are 'not necessarily shared in by every being', as he says. The second (deeper) reason for Space and Time is that no intelligible form of experience is possible without them. They are not properties of experience at all, but necessary conditions for experience. Lotze muddles these so-called 'empirical' and 'transcendental' derivations of Space and bizarrely concludes that it is useless to explain perception by maps in the brain. We have to look for some representation of Space that is not *in itself* spatial; and this is how he arrived at his idea that every nerve fibre coming from the retina carries its own 'local sign', like a postcode, which says what part of the retina it comes from.

The problems are obvious. A postcode is useless without a map. In London, postal district N19 (Upper Holloway) is not geographically between N18 and N20, but is alphabetically nineteenth in the list of northern districts. To use a postcode we have to have a way of decoding into it into a spatial location, and the more we do so, the more and more the representation looks like a map. When it came to it, even Lotze had to agree that his 'local signs' had to be like positions in a map if they were to be of any use. He compares sending a message from the eye to the brain to moving furniture from one house to another. We do not have to place the furniture in the van in the same positions in space as they had in the old house, or in the same positions as we wish them to occupy in the new house; we need only attach a label to each item saying 'kitchen' or 'bedroom no. 1'. Even better, we could number the positions in the new house with some sort of grid, like the grid on an Ordnance Survey map, and put a label on each bit of furniture with its grid reference.

Lotze's two-house analogy presupposes the reassembly of the furniture items into a new spatial order. He has not succeeded in his aim of removing space altogether from the equation. But he was correct in his intuition that the spatial layout of the image on the retina is reassembled into maps in the brain. A simple example to start with is the frog. It is late February and my garden pond is full of jostling amphibians, keen to put their genes into tadpoles. Some have stayed in the pond over winter; others have made long journeys from nearby gardens, where they hibernated under garden refuse or under logs. In summer the frogs sit motionless on the poolside and wait for an insect to alight or fly past; they then strike faster than our eye can see with their tongue at the precise location of the insect. At night they hunt slugs and small insects. We have a pretty good idea how they do it.

A celebrated paper entitled 'What the frog's eye tells the frog's brain', in the *Proceedings of the Institute of Radio Engineers* (1959), said that the frog's eye contains specialised 'bug detectors' for signalling the presence of moving black spots against a white background. Each nerve cell in the frog retina connects not to a single cone but to several over an area of the retinal image called its 'receptive field'. If all the cones had the same effect on the cell, this would not be particularly interesting, but in fact cones in the centre of the receptive field cause the cell to *decrease* its rate of firing while the surrounding cones cause it to *increase*. The net effect, if the whole of the receptive field is stimulated with a large white spot, is that the nerve cell shows little response. What we have here is a tiny analogue computer that is comparing (subtracting) the light falling in the 'plus' region of its receptive field with the light falling in its 'minus'. If a small black object flies into the receptive field it destroys the stand-off between the plus and minus parts of the field and the cell fires. 'Receptive fields' are one of the brain's great inventions, repeated like all good inventions over and over again, not just in vision, but in touch, hearing and smell. The key idea in every case is the same: to compare and contrast sensory signals, rather than transmitting their absolute values. A rough analogy is that we speak the language of 'difference signals' when we track share prices (+2.6), or learn that a football team is three points clear at the top of the League from its nearest rival.

The 'bug detector' in the retina does not solve the problem of telling the frog *where* the bug is. For this, the frog needs some kind of map. The frog eye connects with a part of their brain, called the optic tectum ('roof'), which is a sheet of cells covering the middle part of the brain. A nearby region of the brain in people is involved in controlling the size of the pupil and other eye movements. The map in the frog tectum is orderly (see figure 2.2). Fibres from the part of the retina nearest the frog's nose terminate in the rear of the map and fibres from the rear of the eye terminate in the front of the map. This gives one dimension to the map, like lines of longitude on a chart. The second dimension (latitude) is projected on the axis running at right angles to the first. Fibres from the top of the retina project to the part of each tectum nearest to the midline of the brain; fibres from the bottom of the retina project to the outermost part of the tectum. What this means is that if

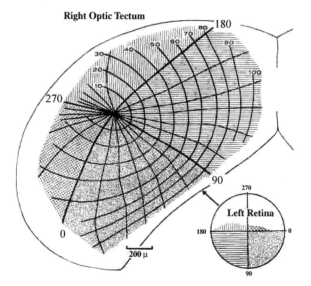

Figure 2.2 The map of the frog's left eye in the right optic tectum

a particular part of the tectal map is activated by a light ray striking the retina, the frog has all the information it needs to work out the direction in space from which the light ray originated.

Curiously, the left-hand side of the frog's visual field is represented in a map in the right-hand side of the tectum, and vice versa. The reason for this 'crossing over' is not known, but it is found in many animals, including ourselves. It does not matter, because mirror reversals and rotations do not affect the usefulness of a map. *McArthur's universal corrective map of the world*, published in Australia, shows South at the top of the map and Australia in its – rightly – superior position. With rare exceptions maps reflect the hegemony of the Northern Hemisphere by placing North at the top. Perhaps this is because of the importance of Polaris, the North Star, in navigation at night – navigators oriented towards Polaris, so they put North at the top of their maps; but this is simply a convention, and the brain is free to choose any convention it likes in its own maps, provided that they are orderly.

But how are the orderly connections between eye and tectum formed in the first place, and how does the frog 'work out' the correspondence between position on the map, and the direction of objects in space? The connections are formed by nerve fibres growing from the retina to the tectum, which must know where to go, just like players walking out on to a cricket pitch at the start of a game. The batsmen head for the stumps. The wicketkeeper must know which end to go to – perhaps the gasworks end. The bowler paces out a position from the stumps and makes a mark so as to find that position more easily the next time. Fielders do not head for a particular patch of grass, but for a position relative to other players: 'silly mid-on' is not an absolute position on the pitch but an approximate one, refined relative to the batsman and other fielders. The basic strategies are: going straight to a landmark, going to a position relative to a landmark, and going to a position relative to other players. Any one of these strategies could be used by optic nerve fibres, and all probably are. The only remaining strategy is 'dead reckoning': emerge from pavilion, head 045 degrees and walk for 2 minutes at 4 knots, then stop. Cricketers do not do this, and nor do nerve cells.

The classic experiment on connections of the amphibian eye was done by Nobel prize-winner Roger Sperry at the California Institute of Technology. Sperry cut the optic nerve of a frog, rotated the eye through 180 degrees, and waited for the optic nerve fibres to grow back again into the tectum. Nerve cells in the part of the eye now nearest to the nose grew back into the front part of the tectum, which is exactly what those particular nerve cells had done during normal development. In other words, they took no account of the fact that the eye had been rotated but went back to the same place as before in the tectum. The cricket analogy becomes somewhat tortuous, but it is as if the players were made to go on to the pitch from a dressing room on the other side of the ground from usual. If they oriented by landmarks on the pitch and by each other, they would go to their normal positions. Only if they navigated by dead reckoning would they end up somewhere else. This is why we can rule out dead reckoning as a system of neural navigation.

Because the nerve cells take no account of their new starting positions relative to the frog's head, the map in the tectum is now reversed up–down and left–right relative to the retinal image. The frog is unaware that this has happened and reads the map as before. Like an explorer with a reversed map, or a navigator making the common error of setting a reciprocal course, the frog is all at sea (as it were). It strikes downwards at flies in its upper visual field, and vice versa.

Sperry guessed that chemical signals were responsible for optic nerve fibres finding their correct place in the tectum. Perhaps each nerve fibre carries a different 'molecular signature' and the signature is different for every cell in the tectum. The task of the growing nerve fibre would then be to find the cell in the tectum with the matching molecular signature. Until it found the right match it would keep looking, like a passenger just arrived at an airport and looking for someone holding up the sign 'Mr P. Smith'. When the nerve fibre found the signal that matched its own it would stop further growth and make the connection. Lotze would have been delighted with this idea, for the proposed chemical signals are just like his 'local signs'. The different chemical signals in the different nerve fibres could all be different molecules, or they could contain different *amounts* of the same molecule. Lotze considered this possibility as well. He noted that it would be convenient if the local signs formed some sort of series, like the numbers 1, 2, 3 ... rather than being arbitrary signs such as ♥ ☏ ▲ ⊘ ⊗. The task for the fibre would be to find the target nerve cell with the concentration of the molecule most closely matching its own. The nerve fibre could find its target by the rules of 'hunt the thimble' rather than by thrashing about until it just happened to find its target. If the molecular signal became more like its own, it would be getting 'hot'; if it became less it would be 'cold'.

Chesil Beach in Dorset stretches 29 km from Bridport Harbour to Chesil on Portland Bill. A strong cross-current has sorted pebbles along the beach in order of their size, from large near Chesil to small at Bridport, and smugglers landing on dark nights could tell exactly where they were by the size of the pebbles underfoot. They were navigating like nerve fibres trying to find their way into the tectum. Many molecules are graded like the stones on Chesil Beach and they play a vital role in development, telling the embryo which end is its head and which its tail, and putting the heart on the left-hand side of the body. In the frog retina two molecules known as TOP_{dv} and TOP_{ap} form two graded series at right angles to one another and make a two-dimensional framework for orienteering.

Graded molecules in the retina and tectum are not the only signposts available. Fibres do not wind their way at random into the arm and out again before finally getting to the tectum. There must be signposts along the way. One important way-point is the midline of the body, where the optic nerve fibres have to decide to cross or not to cross from left to right. In the Siamese cat, some of the nerve fibres get this decision wrong, and this is why the cats end up with a squint. None of the optic nerve fibres in the mutant Belgian sheepdog cross the midline, so the left eye projects entirely to the left side of the brain. How the dog sees the world nobody knows, but there is something not quite right, because the dog has abnormal eye movements. Even so, fibres in the mutant Belgian sheepdog still terminate in an orderly map-like arrangement in the brain (albeit on the wrong side), proof that the chemical signals are similar on the two sides of the brain, and that some extra signpost is involved in getting nerve fibres to the correct side. Various proteins have been found with the responsibility of directing traffic at the midline. Optic nerve axons are repelled by 'slit' if they contain another protein called 'robo'. Axons destined to cross the midline do not contain robo and are initially attracted towards the midline, but as soon as they have crossed, their genes producing robo are activated. This mechanism stops the axons from turning back.

In rural Québec in the 1960s a phone call to one house caused the phones in all the neighbours' houses to ring as well; only the pattern of rings told each householder whether the call was for them. A single wire from the exchange went not just to one subscriber but to several. Something like this is true in the early wiring of the tectum: each nerve cell in the retina is connected to many subscribers in the tectum. The chemical signals that guide nerves to their destination are not sufficiently precise to specify a one-to-one connection. When they first meet the tectum, individual nerve fibres branch out in all directions like a growing tree, to make contact with many nerve cells. (Scientists call these initial connections 'exuberant', which gives a good idea of how much fun to expect at a laboratory party.) Later in development, many of the connections commit suicide, leaving a more precise mapping of points on the retina to points on the map.

In other words, the pruning of wrong connections is just as important as the forming of the correct ones. One idea is that wrong connections are eliminated by applying a simple rule: nerve fibres starting out from neighbouring points on the retina must terminate on neighbouring points in the brain. 'Follow your neighbour' is a good way of keeping a group of children together in a crocodile; but how is this rule enforced in the case of nerve connections? A clue comes from experiments that prevented nerve cells in the retina from firing, using chemicals that blocked the transmission of signals at synapses. Deprived of stimulation, the maps in the tectum remained diffuse and unrefined. The same was true if the frogs were reared under rapid stroboscopic lights, which caused all the nerve cells in the retina to fire at the same instant, suggesting that something about the timing of nerve cells is important in establishing the map of the retina on the tectum. The mechanism seems to be as follows: if the nerve impulses in two nerve fibres are marching in step, like pedestrians on a bridge, they strengthen one another's connections on to the same cell in the tectum; if they are marching out of step, they mutually weaken their connections on the same nerve cell. The weakened connections eventually die, like the twigs on a dying tree.

Put this book down for a moment and look around the room. Try to concentrate on the patches of colour and light that make up the scene, not on familiar objects. Unless you live in a very strange place, you will find your sensations are composed, like a jigsaw puzzle, of interlocking pieces, each of particular colour or brightness. To assemble a jigsaw we look for pieces that resemble one another, like bits of sky or bits of a red dress. A jigsaw composed of random patches of colour is much harder to put together. The earliest jigsaws from the mid-eighteenth century were themselves maps that had been cut into pieces, like that of the London engraver John Spilsbury (1766). His piece containing 'The German or Northsea', for example, is all of the same colour, as it pretty much is in reality – which is a great help to the infant mapmaker.

In typical images, as in jigsaws, nearby points of light have similar brightness and colour. Mathematicians say that neighbouring points of normal images are highly *correlated*, like the colour of scarves at a football match. This means that two nerve fibres coming from neighbouring points on the retina will tend to fire together as the eye moves about a normal scene. Fibres coming from points far apart on the retina will tend to be singing from different hymn sheets, and should not end in the same positions in the brain map. 'Prune' nerve fibres that are singing a different tune from their neighbours, and *voilà*: you have a mechanism for making a topographic map.

The 'neighbourhood' rule would not necessarily work in a different environment from our own. To defeat the rule, scientists have created the Planet Zarg, covered by a dense and perpetual blizzard, illuminated by the occasional enormous flash of lightning. Frogs on Planet Zarg never develop a precise map between retina and tectum; and indeed, why would they need one? The world is the same looking in every direction. One version of Planet Zarg uses a stroboscope to mimic lightning. The strobe makes all the fibres fire at the same time, no matter how distant they are, thus destroying the correlation principle. By imposing a very high correlation between all points on the retina, the stroboscope prevents normal development. What about an animal raised entirely in the dark, like the human foetus? A reasonable guess would be that a precise map fails to develop. But a nice idea (not yet proven) is that the retina overcomes this problem itself, by generating its own spontaneous waves of electrical activity. These waves mimic the correlations found in natural images. If this idea is true, the womb is a virtual reality environment for the nine months of our development.

A map is no good if it cannot be read. R. V. Jones, the author of *Most Secret War* tells the story of a crate that arrived in his workplace bearing the legend: 'Caution! The equipment in this crate is packed in a different manner from that formerly used. Compared with the old methods the equipment is now packed upside down, and the crate must therefore be opened from the bottom. To prevent confusion, the bottom has been labelled "Top".' Language, it seems, is not the ideal way to describe space. The frog does not have this problem. In fact, the frog does not have to 'read' its map at all. It uses its map to catch flies and worms. In theory, the frog could translate the information in its tectal map into a symbolic form – 'Fly at bearing 042 degrees' – using some other brain area, and then send this signal to yet another area of the brain that decodes it into muscular movements. But why not eliminate the middleman, in the interests of speed?

Amphibians do indeed catch their prey without the help of a useless non-spatial entrepreneur. When salamanders spot a worm-like object moving in their field of view, they first move their head to point directly at the object. They then creep forward towards the object until they are close enough to strike. The salamander's brain must have some means of translating the direction of the object in its visual map into an appropriate turning movement of the head. Just underneath the visual map is a second map called the 'pre-motor' map. Points in the visual map are connected directly to the points underneath in the pre-motor map. The pre-motor map contains nerve cells connected directly to the spinal cord, where they make contact with the nerve cells that directly move the muscles of the neck. A given point in the pre-motor map might contain 30 neurones connecting to one muscle (call it 'L') and 50 connecting to a different muscle ('R'). The proportion 30:50 will cause the muscles to move the head in the direction required. Once again, there is no 'middleman' reading the map in the tectum.

Frogs and salamanders tell us that maps exist in the brain, and that they can be directly translated into action. The maps do not have to be first translated into some mysterious non-spatial representation. But perhaps this tells us nothing about our own perception. Frogs and salamanders may be completely unconscious automata, without any awareness of space – as Descartes argued. After all, it is possible to make convincing mechanical automata, like Jacques de Vaucanson's eighteenth-century mechanical duck that flapped its wings, ate real grain and excreted on the table. The mechanical duck had over 1000 moving parts, a very small number compared to the nerve cells of a frog. Perhaps frog prey-catching is a mere unconscious reflex, and maps are useful for reflexes and nothing more; but in the next chapter we shall look at maps in the human brain and see that they are just as important to us as they are to frogs.

3

'The long agitated question'

The defeat of the Russians at Port Arthur in 1904 was one of the seismic events of the twentieth century, signalling the beginning of the end of European imperialism in the East, a process completed by the defeat of the British at Singapore in 1942 and the French at Dien Bien Phu in 1954. It was during the Russian–Japanese war that a young Japanese physician was to make the first detailed drawings of the visual map in the 'occipital lobe' at the back of our head. Most of our knowledge of maps in the human brain has come from the tragedies of disease or injury, and the map of the retina at the back of the brain is no exception.

The surface of the human brain is criss-crossed with deep fissures like crevasses in an ice field. The largest is the vertical one that divides the brain into the left and right cerebral hemispheres. Another obvious cleft is seen on the inner surface of each hemisphere, near to the back: the 'calcarine fissure'. If you wear a glove and put out your hand palm downwards, your hand has the same orientation as the calcarine fissure, and the material of the glove corresponds to the thin rind of grey matter containing the cells of the primary visual cortex – the terminus of the fibres of the optic tract. The top of the glove is the upper lip of the calcarine fissure and the bottom is the lower lip. This thin covering on the top and bottom banks of the fissure – the sides of a crevasse – is where the messages from the retina stop over on a complex march that will eventually take them to over half the brain's surface. It is here, in the primary visual cortex, that the nerve fibres from the two eyes mingle to form a single map.

If we look at a scene first through one eye and then through the other, we shall find that the two views are very similar. There are small differences, certainly: as Leonardo da Vinci knew, the right eye sees more of the world behind us to the right than does the left eye to the left, and an object hidden behind another in one eye may be visible in the other. Even so, our conscious experience through the two eyes is mostly identical. It is as if the left and right eyes form a single map in the brain, and in the first edition of *Optics* Newton (1704) shows us how this might be done. Nerve fibres from the left-hand side of the left eye go to the left-hand side of the brain, without crossing the midline. There they meet fibres from the left-hand side of the right eye, which have crossed the midline. In this way, said Newton, the 'fibres make but one entire Species or Picture'. The crossing over of fibres from the side of each retina nearest to the nose occurs at the χ-shaped optic chiasm. We can predict from Newton's diagram that some brain-damaged patients will be blind in the left-hand side of space through the left eye, and the right-hand side of space through the right eye. Their optic chiasm has been cut in half, preventing nerve fibres from crossing over to the opposite side of the brain. Like fish with eyes on the sides of their head, these patients see different pictures through their two eyes.

How Newton arrived at this theory no one knows, but his inspired guess was supported in 1824 by the English physician and scientist William Hyde Wollaston. Wollaston discovered the elements palladium and rhodium, but more interestingly for us, he suffered from a form of migraine. In his own words:

> It is now more than twenty years since I was first affected with the peculiar state of vision, to which I allude, in consequence of violent exercise I had taken for two or three hours before. I suddenly found that I could see but half the face of a man whom I met; it was the same with respect to every object I looked at. In attempting to read the name JOHNSON, over a door, I saw only SON; the commencement of the name being wholly obliterated from view.

He had became blind in the left half of space. Wollaston's simple but crucial observation was that it did not matter which eye he looked through: the defect was on the left side of space through either eye. Now, he says: 'Since the corresponding points in the two eyes sympathise in disease, their sympathy is evidently from structure, *not from the mere habit of feeling together*.' Wollaston is saying that a learned association between the corresponding parts of the two eyes would be most unlikely to be disrupted by disease; and he suggests instead that there is a map to which both eyes contribute. His new idea was that his migraine knocked out one half of his map (which he locates in a small brain structure called the thalamus). Luckily, his condition was transitory; but he mentions 'a less fortunate acquaintance in which it was permanent. Perhaps this friend had suffered a stroke, permanently damaging one side of the brain.

The first detailed drawing of the visual map at the back of the brain was made by the young Japanese ophthalmologist Tatsuji Inouye, who treated soldiers wounded in the war between the Imperial Russian Army and the Japanese. The head injuries studied by Inouye were caused by the small, high-velocity bullets fired from the new Russian Moisin Nagent rifle. These often made a clear, straight track between entrance and exit wounds, which made it easy for neurologists to see which areas of the brain had been damaged. As he explains, Inouye published his observations in the hope that they would make people realise the terrible destruction that could be wrought by modern weapons: 'The hardship and ferocity of the last war led me to publish these observations. The awfulness and horror of the experience, of which those who did not take part cannot have the slightest appreciation, at the same time raised the hope in me and in all other physicians that in future, war may, if possible be prevented' (*Tatsuji Inouye*, 1908).

A vain hope, as it turned out, of course. Wars continued, and the First World War produced many more cases of blindness from gunshot wounds, confirming Inouye's case histories. Inouye found that localised damage to the back of the brain produced local areas of blindness, which he refered to as 'scotomata'. For example, on the 405th day after injury he measured the extent of Mr Tanaka's field defect along the vertical meridian: 'For that I used small white targets of cotton wool of 6 mm across on the point of a thin instrument of the kind that is used to widen the lachrymal ducts. I moved it repeatedly from the defective side of the visual field towards the fixation point, holding it for 1 s and then suddenly retracting it again. I asked him to say yes when he first noticed the test target . . .' An unusual and oddly touching feature of Inouye's journal is that he never fails to mention the state of the weather. On this occasion, 'The weather is somewhat cloudy'; in another case, 'The weather was beautiful.' The tests were carried out in daylight, the level of which affects visual acuity.

Local damage produced local areas of blindness. For example, damage to the upper lip of the calcarine fissure towards the back of the left hemisphere produced complete blindness in the lower half of the central area of the right visual field, while injury to the back part of the *left* hemisphere produced blindness in the *right* field. The area of blindness is the same whether the patient looks out of the left or the right eye (as in Wollaston's case), which tells us that the inputs from the two eyes mingle in the same parts of the brain.

Inouye put the information from all of his patients together to draw a map around the calcarine fissure (see Figure 3.1). First he plotted the visual field as if the eye were a hemisphere, like a ping-pong ball cut in half. The pole corresponds to the centre of the visual field, where our acuity is highest, and the equator corresponds to the far periphery of our vision. The prime meridian, corresponding to Greenwich on a globe, divides the left visual field (East) from the right (West). Lines of latitude are great circles going from 0 at the pole to 90 degrees at the equator. There is no southern hemisphere, because the retina is treated as a hemisphere rather than a full sphere.

How can we now map this hemisphere on to the two-dimensional banks of the calcarine fissure? The sheet can be unfolded like an Ordnance Survey map, with the main fold corresponding to the bottom of the crevasse. So we are now trying to map a hemisphere on to a flat, two-dimensional sheet. This is the problem faced by any mapmaker trying to map the globe on a flat surface. One familiar solution is the Mercator projection, in which the lines of longitude are drawn parallel, instead of converging at the pole.

Its great disadvantage is that it exaggerates areas near the pole. This is politically incorrect. But exaggerating the polar regions of the eye is not a problem, for there are many more nerve cells in the eye around the pole (the centre of the visual field) than in the same area at the equator (the peripheral visual field). This is why our visual acuity is much higher in the centre of the retina than in the periphery and why we find it hard to read normal-size letters unless we look directly at them. A letter has to be much larger in the peripheral field before we can recognise its shape (see figure 3.2). The area of the brain map devoted to the polar latitudes between 0 and 10 degrees is roughly equal to the whole area devoted to the latitudes 60–90 degrees, despite the hugely greater area of the visual field represented by the latter.

The map of the retina on the brain is democratic. Equal numbers of nerve cells in the retina are represented by roughly equal areas of the brain map. In this respect it is like a voting map in which constituencies are represented by their number of voters, not by their geographical area. For example, in the map of the US Presidential election in 2000

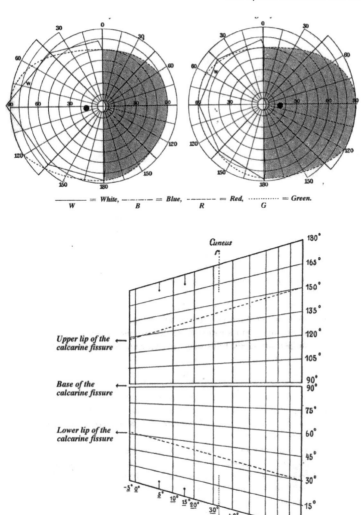

Figure 3.1 The visual fields of Case 2 (U. Takeda, a twenty-four-year-old infantryman wounded at Sha-ho) and Inouye's map. Inouye's map puts the upper visual field on the lower bank of the calcarine fissure and the lower visual field on the upper bank. The gap between the cerebral hemispheres marks the prime meridian, dividing left from right visual field. The bottom of the calcarine fissure marks the 90 degree meridian dividing upper from lower visual field. And finally, the lines of latitude change as we go from the front of the fissure to the back. The centre of the retina (the pole) maps on to the rear of the fissure and spills out on to the back of the brain. The far periphery of the visual field (the equator) is buried deep in the hidden frontmost part of the calcarine fissure. This means that injuries confined to the rearmost tip of the brain produce blindness in the centre of the visual field, sparing the periphery.

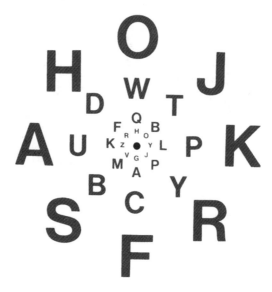

Figure 3.2 Our visual acuity is much higher in the direction of our gaze than in other directions. Acuity decreases dramatically the further away the object is from the centre of the retina. This is illustrated by the Anstis eye chart, in which letters increase in size from the centre so as to be equally readable. If we look in the centre of the chart, we can read all the letters with roughly equal ease, but only because their size increases in proportion to their distance from the centre. When this eye chart is represented on the cortex, each letter would be seen by approximately the same number of nerve cells.

New York State is much larger than Utah because it sends thirty-three votes to the Electoral College, while Utah sends only five.

Neither Inouye's patients nor Wollaston's temporary blindness prove that left and right eyes project to identical parts of the map. They might, for example, project to neighbouring points in the map, but not to the same cells. Colour televisions appear to show a single image from their three coloured projectors, but actually the red, green and blue spots make a pointillist image (in which they can be seen separately under a magnifying glass). Maybe, when looked at hard enough, the left and right eye maps will also remain distinct in the brain. What Wollaston called 'the long agitated question of single vision with two eyes' was not finally settled until the Nobel prize-winning investigations of David Hubel and Thorsten Wiesel in the 1960s and 1970s, in which they used very finely pointed needles to record the electrical activity of single nerve cells in the visual map of anaesthetised cats and monkeys. Their surprising news was that the left and right eye

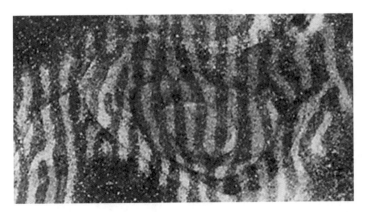

Figure 3.3 Ocular dominance stripes in the visual cortex of the monkey. A radioactive chemical injected into one eye has moved back along the optic nerve to the brain, where it shows up as black stripes, alternating with unstained (white) stripes connected to the uninjected eye.

maps are indeed partly distinct in the brain map, like the colour maps on a TV screen, rather than being completely united. Many of the individual nerve cells they recorded in the map were driven by either one eye or the other, not by both. Looked at from the surface of the brain, the two maps resembled the stripes of a zebra, with white stripes corresponding to the left eye and black stripes to the right (see figure 3.3).

Hubel and Wiesel's map was like the face of a new continent. However, the map in the striate cortex differs from a cartographer's map in one important respect: it is three-dimensional, not flat. The surface of the cerebral hemispheres – the grey matter – is only a few millimetres thick, but this is enough to contain thousands of nerve cells at each point in the map. These cells are organised into distinct layers like a sandwich, one of which was first seen by an Italian medical student at the University of Parma, Francesco Gennari, who published his account in the monograph *De Peculiari Stuctura Cerebri* in 1782. Gennari cut sections of frozen brain and found a thin white stripe, under the surface and running parallel to it. This 'stripe of Gennari' is more marked in the parts of the brain corresponding to the visual area at the back of the brain, or 'striate cortex'. There are six layers in the striate cortex, and the fibres of the optic tract enter layer IV. The layers are further subdivided into sub-layers, and the precise location of Gennari's stripe is layer IVc. Gennari was one of the great neuro-anatomists of all time, but sadly he died impoverished at the age of forty-five, after years of misery, probably brought on in part by compulsive gambling.

In Gennari's stripe all the nerve cells are driven either from the left eye or the right, but in the upper layers of the cake (nearer the surface of the brain) the picture changes. The two maps become more united. Many cells respond equally to stimulation in the left and the right eye, from corresponding places in the two retinal maps. Others respond to both eyes, but have a 'preference' for one eye over the other. Wollaston's 'long agitated question' has been solved. The fibres from the two eyes first of all make two separate maps, intermingled like zebra stripes, but later on they become united into a single map. Apart from the striate cortex, the brain is like Polyphemus the Cyclops, with his single eye.

Like 'bug detectors' in the frog retina, cells in the visual cortex are calculators. They have 'receptive fields', which compare light levels across the image, and calculate difference signals. However, Hubel and Wiesel discovered that the analogue computing powers of single nerve cells in the striate cortex greatly outstrip those in the frog retina. The receptive fields of bug detectors are circular and do not care if the image falling in their receptive field is rotated. Hubel and Wiesel discovered more or less by accident that their cells 'preferred' elongated rectangles to spots of light, and that they responded best to rectangles in particular orientations, for example, vertical rather than horizontal (▌ vs ▬) . The reason for this is that their receptive fields are themselves roughly rectangular in shape: another example of analogue computing. Each cell 'prefers' the image that fits best into its receptive field, and the receptive fields come in every possible combination of size and shape, like locks waiting for the appropriate key to activate them. Other cells prefer lines of a particular tilt moving in a particular direction: they have receptive fields tilted in both space and time. As we shall see later, these analogue computers allow us to perceive motion.

The map is now getting complicated, because each point in it contains cells with their own preferences for eye dominance and for tilt. Hubel and Wiesel found that cells with similar tilt preference formed columns at right angles to the surface of the brain. Within a column the cells have receptive fields in slightly different retinal positions. Neighbouring columns have similar but not identical tilt preferences. If we use colour to represent tilt preference in the striate cortex, we get a beautiful 'pinwheel' map (see plate section). Cells with similar preference for tilt lie along the same arms of the pinwheel, and the preferred angle changes gradually as we go clockwise around the wheel.

All the arms meet together in a 'singularity' at the centre of the wheel, like a black hole in which preferences disappear.

The striate cortex of the monkey is tiled with small areas about 2 sq mm in size, within each of which both eyes and all tilt preferences are represented. Hubel and Wiesel called these tiles 'hypercolumns'. Each hypercolumn is responsible for a different part of the overall topographical map. The roughly 100,000 cells in a hypercolumn form complex connections with one another and with neighbouring hypercolumns; each hypercolumn can be considered as a sophisticated analogue computer, itself composed of smaller analogue devices (the individual nerve cells). The function of the hypercolumn-computer is to begin the analysis of the image, a process that will eventually recognise objects such as faces. Hypercolumns contain the same number of cells, whatever their position in the map. Those in the centre of our visual field give us higher acuity, not because they contain more cells, but because they have the same number of cells as the hypercolumns in the peripheral visual field, which are looking at a much larger area. The relation between hypercolumns and areas on the retina is somewhat like that between constituencies in the British parliamentary elections, which represent hugely unequal areas, but roughly equal numbers of people.

The striate cortex is a map, but a map of a very peculiar kind. Its elements are laid out spatially in a way that corresponds with the retinal image, but they are not points, as they would be in a geographical map. Each point is a complex analogue computer – the hypercolumn. The map in the striate cortex is very different from an image: so different, indeed, that some have doubted whether it can be the place in the brain where visual consciousness arises. Perhaps the striate cortex is just another kind of retina embedded in the brain, and the true seat of visual awareness is in other parts of the brain. Once again, Inouye's patients pointed the way forward to these previously undiscovered regions.

Inouye's Case 2 (U. Takeda, a twenty-four-year-old infantryman, and a farmer in civilian life) had a penetrating wound from a bullet that had entered his right brow and exited through the back of his head on the left, completely destroying the left striate cortex. He was therefore blind in his right visual field, but spared in the left (see figure 3.1). Mr Tanaka had no subjective experience of a small white object in his right visual field, and he did have such experience in his left field; but this does not mean that he saw normally in his left field. For a start, he was unable to read. He had been able to write rather well before the injury: afterwards he was able to write his name with his right hand, correctly but awkwardly, and could write the signs for the Japanese syllables (hiragana). However, if shown the letters that he had written, he was unable to name them. He could name a cup or a book but not most other things. He confused red, green and blue.

Inouye uses the old term *Seelenblindheit* – literally, 'mental blindness' – to describe Mr Tanaka's loss of object recognition. The same condition would nowadays be called 'visual object agnosia'. Inability to name colours is called 'achromatopsia'. Inouye's translators avoid anachronism by using the older term 'apperceptive blindness' from the contemporary English literature. 'Apperception', we are told in the *Oxford Companion to the Mind*, was invented by the philosopher Gottfried Wilhelm von Leibniz (1646–1716) as a way of distinguishing passive perception from the understanding of what we see. An object like a cup might be sensed as a white object having a particular outline, without our having any knowledge that it is an object called a 'cup' or that it is used for drinking tea. We might, in other words, perceive an object in our visual field, without having the *apperception* that it is a cup.

Bertrand Russell credited Leibniz with having made the distinction between unconscious and conscious perception. We are having perceptions all the time, says Leibniz, even during sleep and (in the extreme case) death, but only in fully conscious states of mind are we aware of having perceptions. The latter is the apperceptive state.

Apperception figures prominently in Kant's *Critique of Pure Reason*, where the philosopher sets himself the task of showing that observers could have the experience of different perceptions belonging to *them*, only if perceptions happened in Space and Time. In other words, it would not be possible to see a red tomato unless the redness and the tomato-ness were somehow put together in a medium called 'Space', and a tomato in one place could be distinct from an apple in the same place only if we have Time. 'Anon' has put this more clearly: 'Time prevents all bad things happening at once; Space stops them all happening to you.'

Inouye speculates that the *Seelenblindheit* of his case Mr Tanaka was caused by extensive brain damage to regions of the brain outside the striate cortex but surrounding it. He says:

The total visual area I think can be described functionally as consisting of two parts which I should like to call the principal visual area and the neighbouring visual area. The principal visual area up till now has simply been refered to as the visual cortex in which a precise projection in the sense of a copy of the retina on the cortex has taken place. The neighbouring visual areas include the remaining visual area where there is still a projection but not a precise one.

Inouye's map has served later explorers well. The *terra incognita* surrounding the primary visual cortex has been mapped in minute detail, to an extent undreamed of by Inouye himself. Anatomists have many techniques at their disposal for unravelling the wiring of the most complicated machine on the planet. One is based on the 'use it or lose it' principle. If a small area of the brain is damaged, the nerve fibres connecting it to other areas no longer carry traffic, and they degenerate. Special stains pick out these degenerating fibres, betraying the areas to which they connect. The technique reveals connections between Inouye's 'principal visual area', now called V1 and other areas surrounding it, and the functions of these areas can then be investigated by recording from the cells there. For example, Semir Zeki at University College London showed that the area called 'V5' contained cells that responded particularly vigorously to moving stimuli. Further discoveries followed quickly. If we had been able to follow the spread of known 'V' areas on a coloured map, we should have seen vision spreading like an empire, until almost one half of the monkey cortex had been occupied. The empire includes much of the parietal lobe and temporal lobes, as well as the occipital lobe (see plate section).

The area immediately surrounding V1 on either side of the calcarine fissure is called V2. A peculiarity of V2 is that it is necessarily in two entirely separated parts, above and below the calcarine fissure, corresponding to the upper and lower parts of the visual field. The two halves of the map are connected by nerve fibres that run between the two cerebral hemispheres across a huge connecting cable: the corpus callosum. Within its two halves, V2 has a recognisable map of the visual field not unlike that of V1, but, as Inouye guessed, the map is less precise. Each of the cells in V2 has a large receptive field, which means that it looks at a large area of the retina. The other V areas spread over the surface of the brain in all directions, some going downwards towards the temporal lobe and others upwards towards the parietal lobe. Zeki found that the majority of cells in area V4 have preferences for the colour of the stimulus in their part of the map. This is different from the situation in V1, where only some cells have colour preferences.

Cells in V5, on the other hand, have much stronger preferences for motion than for colour (although some colour preference exists as well). Again, motion preference is not unique to V5: it exists in V1 as well, but not in all cells.

It is time to take some bearings. Why should there be these multiple maps? Why are there any maps at all? And what is the connection between these maps and our experience of Space? A clue to the function of maps lies in the frog's tectum. The frog's retina is mapped directly on to the upper layers of the tectum, and this map is in turn connected to a pre-motor map beneath, allowing the frog to orient towards its prey. This whole system is an analogue computer, in which space has a continuous representation from input to output; but the computer works only because of the orderly mapping. Imagine the problems if the points in the pre-motor map bore only a random relation to directions in space. Each nerve cell in the upper tectal map would now have to find its way to an arbitrary nerve cell in the pre-motor map, rather than to its immediate neighbour in the downstairs flat. This might just conceivably be achieved by some immensely complicated genetic program. Learning by trial and error might also succeed in the long run, but, as the economist J. M. Keynes was fond of saying, in the long run we shall all be dead.

There is a deeper problem with random wiring. The frog's eye is no more perfect than our own, and flies and worms are satisfyingly large. As a result, the prey projects a blurred image that covers the receptive fields of many nerve cells. If these cells were randomly scattered over the tectum (rather than being in a tight group) and if each projected to a random point in the pre-motor map, the wiring would have to be quite incredibly precise. Each cell in the retina would have to project to one cell in the tectum, which would in turn have to project to one point in the pre-motor map. Even if a cell connected not only with its correct partner but with the neighbours on either side, complete confusion would result. Neighbours in the pre-motor map would issue entirely contradictory commands to the motor map: the head would be paralysed, like an army given conflicting orders from the General Staff.

This nightmare is avoided by the analogue map of the frog's tectum. So long as neighbouring cells in the pre-motor map cause similar head movements, a group of them can be activated without causing conflict. Paradoxically, a rough analogue map avoids the need for precise one-to-one wiring. The frog moves its head in response to orders not from a single cell, but from many: a so-called 'population code'. A population code is one in which each nerve cell in a large collection 'votes' for a particular outcome, and the final vote takes every cell into account. In a parliamentary election this would correspond to proportional representation rather than first-past-the-post; but this voting system will only work for the frog if neighbouring cells in the map vote in roughly the same way, as human neighbours tend to do in elections.

Voting systems are also at work in our own brain, controlling the movements of our eyes. Good tricks tend to be copied in evolution, and analogue maps are widespread. The powerhouse for our eye movements lies in a region of the midbrain called the superior colliculus (little hill). As in the frog's tectum (from which it evolved), this structure consists of several layers, with a map of the retina at the top. Stimulation of deeper layers causes movements of the eyes in a direction that depends on which part of the map is stimulated. Movements in similar directions are caused by stimulation of neighbouring parts of the map, and if two parts of the map are stimulated at the same time, the eyes move along a path that is the average of the two. The system is, it seems, another analogue computing machine, based on a map.

Why are there so many different maps in the brain, instead of a single master map? The answer, as Semir Zeki cogently argues in his book *A Vision of the Brain*, is that brain maps are not passive images, but active machines for carrying out different activities. Analogue computers are good at doing what they do, but they do only the one thing. The computer that moves the eyes is not adapted to recognising faces, or even colour. As a result, patients with one kind of brain injury can completely lose the ability to see colour, without having any problems with eye movements. The eye-control computer is colour-blind, and colour is analysed in a quite different part of the brain. Proliferation of special-purpose computers may seem wasteful, but there are even more nerve cells in the brain of the American President than there are dollars in his entire military budget. Our brain can get away with using special-purpose analogue systems because it has many of them. There are 10 thousand million cells in human grey matter alone, and 60 million million connections between them. This does not even include the cerebellum, where a single Purkinje cell can make up to *two hundred thousand* connections with incoming nerve fibres. With this massive machinery at its disposal the brain can afford to have large numbers of specialised analogue devices devoted to different tasks, which can be carried out at the same time, or, as engineers say, 'in parallel'. This allows the brain to overcome the slowness of its components. Nerve fibres fire at a maximum rate of a thousand times per second, compared to the one hundred million or so operations per second of a Pentium microprocessor. The slowness of the brain would be a devastating disadvantage, if it were not for the fact that millions of nerve cells can be active at the same time, performing different computations. What nerve cells lack in speed, they make up for by quantity.

The next chapter will describe how the brain also contains many specialised systems for dealing with the third dimension in its maps of space. As Bishop Berkeley told us, light rays arriving at the eye do not directly tell us how far they have travelled. So how can we tell the three-dimensional shape of objects, and how can we tell how far they are away? The answer to these two questions (shape and range) turns out to be somewhat different. There is no master 3-D map of the world in the brain, only the usual messy democracy of voters.

4

Cyclopean Vision

The walls of Tyrins, on the edge of the Argolic Gulf, are 7 metres thick. In Greek legend these, and the nearby fortress of Mycenae, were built by the race descended from the Cyclops (hence the architectural term 'Cyclopean' for 'huge or massive'). Like the architects of the 1960s, the builders of Mycenae were louts, but they had good three-dimensional vision. Polyphemus, the most famous of his homicidal and gloomy race, could deal impressively and destructively with moving objects: 'Neither reply nor pity came from him, but in one stride he clutched at my companions and caught two in his hands like squirming puppies to beat their brains out, spattering the floor.' Polyphemus had only one eye, in the centre of his forehead. So how did he see the third dimension? Everyone knows that two eyes are needed to see properly in three dimensions, yet here is a Cyclops creating havoc amongst the binocularly gifted. The *Odyssey* does not once mention Polyphemus' single eye as a disadvantage.

The idea that we need two eyes to see the world in three dimensions is a delusion. There have been one-eyed test cricketers, cyclopean pirates, and at least one excellent monocular admiral. Two eyes do not help a pilot to land on an aircraft carrier, and in spite of all the propaganda from the vendors of 3-D postcards and movies, the absence of depth in ordinary paintings, photographs and films does not cause them to be perceived as flat. The surface of the paint and canvas looks flat, but the scene depicted *through* the surface is seen as three-dimensional. If all surface structure is removed, as when we examine a colour slide through a back-lit slide viewer, the ambiguity is resolved and we see only the depth.

Like many after him, Bishop Berkeley mistakenly thought that the problem for 3-D vision was to measure distance. Light rays coming from an object carry no clue to how far they have travelled; hence the problem. We can call this the problem of measuring range, because in the man-made world it is the job of rangefinders. Rangefinders work on the principle that if we know the angle of an object from two points a known distance apart, we can calculate its distance. This is how astronomers measure the distance to the nearest stars, using the diameter of the Earth's orbit around the Sun as a baseline. An early military rangefinding device called the Watkin mekometer (see figure 4.1) used two soldiers tied together with string as its observing platform. One observer pointed directly to the distant object and the other measured its angle though a telescope. The mekometer was used in the Boer War, but alas, the crafty Boers soon learned the length of the string, and by measuring its apparent size, they calculated the range of the observers and turned the tables upon them.

Figure 4.1 The Watkin mekometer, used for rangefinding in the Boer war. The string was of known length and at right angles to one of the two observers, allowing range to be calculated from the angle of the target to the second observer. Unfortunately, the Boers found out the length of the string, and used its apparent size to calculate the range of the mekometer.

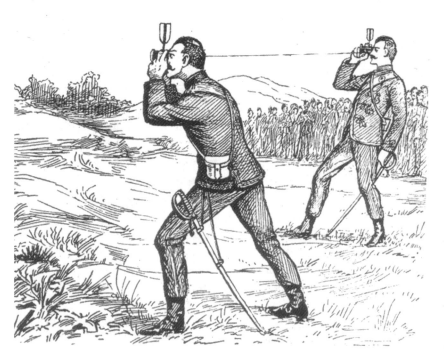

The next generation of rangefinders used prisms and mirrors instead of two observers. These allowed the observer to superimpose the image of an object from two vantage points and to measure the angle between them by bringing them into register. It is easy to make an analogy between the soldiers of the mekometer and the two eyes in our head, and indeed, chameleons do use the angle between their eyes to measure range when striking at prey with their tongue. Their eyes swivel around in their sockets like ballbearings in a socket, and the chameleon can sense their position well enough to determine range. We do the same to some extent. If we cross our eyes to fuse the images of two pennies on a table into a single percept, the penny looks nearer than it actually is, and in consequence looks smaller. This method of estimating range is only very crude, however. Experiments show that our brains do not know the exact positions of our eyes well enough to estimate distances beyond a few feet. We are in the position of the early Greek astronomers, who failed to find the distance of the Sun from the Earth because the angles were just too small for them to measure.

In fact, we do not need two eyes at all to see the third dimension. If we did, movies and paintings would look like cardboard cut-outs and be dismal failures. On the contrary, they convey a vivid impression of solid objects. We may not be able to estimate range from paintings, but they do not look flat. The problem of seeing depth is not the same as that of calculating range, and the reason for this is that range is only one of many kinds of information about depth. Although the image is flat, it is rich in information, which our brains exploit to the full. We can observe many of these clues to the third dimension in paintings – for example, in Sebastien Stoskopff's still life *Les Cinq Sens* (The Five Senses), shown in the plate section.

The Five Senses is part of the collection in the Musée des Beaux Arts attached to Strasbourg Cathedral. The same collection contains Stoskopff's *Corbeille de Verres*, in which the three-dimensional shape of glasses is indicated almost entirely by reflections. *The Five Senses* was painted in 1633. According to the museum catalogue, smell is represented by the vase of flowers, touch by the dice on the chessboard, hearing by the several musical instruments, taste by the bowl of fruit, and vision by the Black Dog (this is as obvious as an allegory on the banks of the Nile).

Seven ways of representing depth are easily identifiable in *The Five Senses*:

Shape from shading. The globe, the vase and the young woman's neck are shadowed on the right, indicating a light source from the left (which agrees with the shadowing of the violin on the wall and the shadow under the open music book, a Protestant transcription of Psalm 76). Assuming that light is coming from the left, we can interpret the sequence of foldings along the tablecloth (from left to right) as a convexity, followed by a concavity. 'Shape from shading' is one of the tricks that give purely digital movies such as *Toy Story* their stunning realism. If we know where the light is coming from, we can calculate the pattern of shading in the image, even if the objects are completely imaginary. Computer graphics artists call this a 'lighting model'.

Unfortunately, a lighting model cannot always be run in reverse. As for many algorithms – mathematical rules that can be slavishly applied – we cannot work backwards from shading to 3-D shape. If we know the numbers of votes cast for each party in each constituency of the General Election, we can calculate the numbers of MPs of each party in the new Parliament; but the calculation cannot be reversed. Similarly, if we observe a pattern of shading on an object in the image, we cannot infer both the lighting and the shape of the object: there are two pieces of information (lighting and shape) in the three-dimensional world and only one (shading) in the image. Infinite combinations of lighting and shape can produce the same image, and we can infer shape from shading only if we have evidence about the source of the light or if we make assumptions about it. Sometimes the position of the light source is given away by a direct reflection from a mirror or glass, but there is no obvious example of this 'specular reflection' in *The Five Senses*. When there is no evidence, we have to rely on assumptions (such as that illumination comes from above, as we saw in the earlier example of the mounds and craters (see figure 1.4)). This assumption is overridden in *The Five Senses*, in part because we know that the scene is indoors.

The relationship between shadows and shape is subtle, and not always intuitively obvious. For example, one might think that the shadows of all the objects in a scene should point in the same direction, if the scene is lit by a single light source such as the sun. But no: the direction of a shadow depends on the angle of the surface on to which it is projected. In Luca Signorelli's *Flagellation of Christ*, a figure on the right of the painting casts a different shadow from each of his two legs (see plate section). One is tempted at first to think that this is a mistake, but experiment proves otherwise. The shadows of the two legs must meet at the shadow of the torso, so the 'V' shape is inevitable.

Perspective. In *The Five Senses* the distorted squares of the chessboard tell the viewer that the surface is slanting away from the viewpoint. The curving lines on the lute betray its shape. The door on the right of the wall safe is a parallelogram to indicate that it is opening outwards. The safe is recessed within a copper frame (according to the catalogue). Or is the safe coming out from the wall? Could 'the wall safe' even be only a trompe l'oeil, painted on the far wall to deceive the eye and reproduced faithfully in Stoskopff's image? Impossible to tell from the evidence: one has to know what the real shape is to start with. Shape on the retina, or in a painting, is inherently ambiguous, because infinitely many three-dimensional scenes can project to the same image. Constellations like the Great Bear (the Dipper) are simply shapes produced by chance from stars that have nothing to do with one another. Like shape from shading, perspective can suggest three-dimensional shape, but only if we make assumptions.

Texture. The squares on the chessboard decrease systematically in size from the bottom of the board to the top. This indicates depth because nearer objects cast larger images on the retina than those further away. Texture gradients can be seen in receding tiled floors, in the stones on gravel paths and in vegetation. They cause a powerful impression of depth in their own right, and are used as such in many works of op art.

Occlusion. We can see Psalm 76 on top of the lute but not the lute through the psalm. The lute in turn interrupts our view of the table-cloth. The hair of the young woman interrupts a vertical line on the wall behind. If the image of one object is interrupted by another, we see the interrupted object as further away. Once again, this interpretation depends on an assumption: that straight lines with gaps in them belong to the same object. So powerful is this assumption that we make it even when there is no other evidence for an object in front. We see so-called 'cognitive contours' in front of an interrupted cube, even though the light intensity of the 'bars' is the same as that of the background (see figure 4.2).

The upwards-sloping ground-plane. As Berkeley knew, we have to move our eyes downwards to see our feet, and upwards to see the clouds

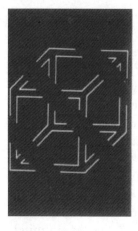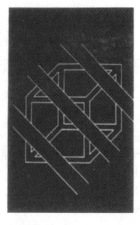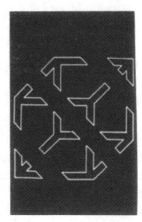

Figure 4.2 Gregory's occluded Necker cube. The left-hand image will be seen by most viewers as a cube, partly visible through a fence of diagonal bars. The bars have the same luminance as the rest of the page, and would be completely invisible if the cube fragments were removed. With some effort the cube can be made to 'flip' in the third dimension, illustrating the ambiguity of perspective. In the image on the right the cube fragments have been made into closed contours, and for most viewers the cube vanishes. The white lines surrounding the closed fragments are inconsistent with the assumption of occluding black bars.

in the sky. The rule that distant objects are projected to higher points in the image is preserved in many paintings, and is the main rule used by young children to indicate distance in their drawings. In *The Five Senses*, the lowest point in the image, and also the nearest, is the tablecloth. The distant figure on the outdoor terrace is about halfway up the picture, and above her are the more distant hills. The rule admits many exceptions. The young woman's face is higher in the image plane than the hills, because she is tall and near. We can infer nothing about distance from the fact that the top of the wall safe is higher than the violin.

Familiar size. The image of the woman on the terrace is tiny in comparison to the young woman in the foreground. Either she is a midget or she is far away. If we assume that she is of normal size, we can infer that she is far away. The problem with this reasoning is that it can become circular. We infer that the woman is far away because her image is small, but we infer that she is of normal size (despite her small image) because she is seen as distant. Psychologists call the latter form of inference 'size constancy', but saying that things are seen as the same size because of 'size constancy' is like explaining the powers of opium by a 'somniferic principle'. Exactly this problem has arisen in explaining the 'harvest moon' illusion. The astronomer and mathematician Ptolemy commented on the fact that the Moon on the horizon looks considerably larger than the Moon at its zenith. A much-canvassed explanation is that the Moon on the horizon is judged to be distant because it is seen behind trees or houses, and it is therefore expanded by 'size constancy'. However, most people think that the horizon Moon appears *nearer* than the Moon at the zenith, and this has been explained by its appearing larger!

Atmospheric perspective. Distant trees and mountains become indistinct and become more blue, as the short wavelength light is scattered more than red.

The one-eyed Polyphemus therefore had no shortage of information about his three-dimensional world, but he had another kind of information even more powerful than the cues in *The Five Senses*: he could move about and observe the result on his retina. If we lie down under a tree and look upwards into the canopy with one eye shut, it looks oddly flat. To see the canopy in its full glory, move the head from side to side through a distance of about 30cm at a rate of about one oscillation per second. The impression of volume in the tree emerges like a developing photograph in the darkroom. We have observed *motion parallax*: the different appearance of a three-dimensional scene seen from different vantage points. When the head is moved, the relative positions of leaves and branches at different distances change. The images of nearer objects on the retina move through a greater angle than the images of further objects. We use this relative movement in the image as a powerful source of information about shape and range.

Like other cues to depth, motion parallax depends on assumptions, and when these are invalid we experience strange effects. One such was noticed by Ernst Mach, the physicist who invented Mach numbers to measure the speed of sound, and first suggested that the visual system contains analogue computers for comparing light at different parts of the image. The illusion called 'Mach's card' is simply a birthday or other greetings card, preferably with no writing on its inside faces, and placed on the table so that it is viewed from inside (see figure 4.3d). If one eye is covered and the card stared at intently for a minute or so without moving the eyes, it will eventually appear to 'flip' in the third dimension so that its nearer, convex fold now appears concave and

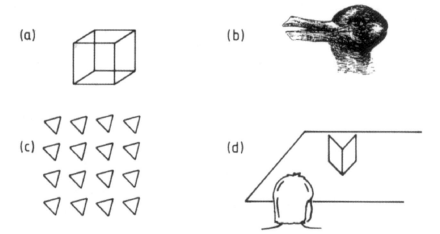

Figure 4.3 Perceptually ambiguous figures: (a) the Necker cube (b) Jastrow's duck- rabbit (c) Attneave's flying triangles (d) Mach's card

pointing away from the eye. The two-dimensional projection of the image on the retina is insufficient to distinguish between pointing-towards and pointing-away, and eventually we oscillate like Buridan's ass between the two alternatives. If we wait until we see the card in the 'wrong' direction and then move our head from side to side, the card appears to rotate around its own axis in time with the motion.

The delusions of the paranoid follow one another with mad but logical inevitability. If you advise a person suffering from paranoia that the neighbour is not really conspiring against him with the assistance of an X-ray machine hidden in the food mixer, you cease to be a solution and become a part of the problem. Something like this is happening in our brain with Mach's card. Our visual brain assumes that the far edge of the card is pointing towards us, rather than away. When we move our head the motion parallax is inconsistent with this assumption, unless we further assume that the card has really moved, so for a moment at least we see the card as moving in exact synchrony with our head.

Movement parallax is powerful, but it may not always be a good idea to attract attention to oneself by moving about. An alternative to movement is to compare the different images in the two eyes: another form of parallax. The first person to demonstrate that the brain does use the parallax between the eyes was the physicist Charles Wheatstone, who used a simple arrangement of mirrors to present line drawings of simple objects separately to the two eyes. The left and right eye pictures were drawn from slightly different viewpoints. His invention became the basis for the 'parlour stereoscope', the device that enchanted Victorians with the sensation of 'stereopsis' – literally, 'solid vision'. It fitted in wonderfully with the other Victorian enthusiasms for the Empire and for the sublime: here were all those exotic places and subjects of the Queen to be wondered at, and all those beetling crags.

As nearly always happens with new inventions, the stereoscope was rapidly followed by claims that it had been discovered before. The Scottish physicist and inventor Sir David Brewster was unable to believe that Wheatstone and not he had thought of the device first, and pushed the claims of various obscure rivals, on the ABW principle – Anyone But Wheatstone. In *The Times* of 15 October 1856 Brewster (hiding behind the pseudonym 'A') claimed that the stereoscope was the 'invention of Mr James Elliot, teacher of Mathematics in Edinburgh, who contrived it in 1834 but did not execute it till 1839'. To this, Wheatstone made the acid reply:

Sir: D. Brewster and your correspondent, in accordance with him, represent Mr. Elliot as having conceived the idea of the stereoscope in 1834, and as having realised his conception in 1839. Admitting these dates, the first is the year after my experiments had been announced in a work of standard authority, and the latter date is the year after my instrument had been completely described and extensively known. It moreover appears that Mr. Elliot made no public announcement of what he is stated to have done until 18 years after the public were informed of my results. (*The Times*, 18 October 1856)

Brewster patented the prismatic version of the stereoscope that proved much less bulky and more convenient than Wheatstone's mirror version. He also patented the kaleidoscope. Wheatstone, on the other hand, invented the concertina and the Wheatstone bridge. Honours were even, in retrospect.

The stereoscope put it beyond doubt that binocular parallax can give rise to an impression of the third dimension entirely by itself. One advantage of binocular parallax is its very high precision. The smallest differences in distance that we can discern when using two eyes correspond to the thickness of a sheet of ordinary typing paper viewed at a distance of about 10 metres. This at first sight seems impossible, because the equivalent parallax on the retina corresponds to only one tenth of the size of a single cone. Like the flight of the bumblebee, the acuity of the human eye seems to defy explanation, but the brain achieves the apparently impossible by special-purpose analogue computers that compare the images in the two eyes. These analogue devices are nerve cells that are connected to both eyes.

These 'binocular' nerve cells compare the amount of light falling in their receptive fields in the two eyes. Parallax causes a difference between the two eyes, which the single cell can detect. One binocular cell by itself cannot distinguish real parallax from other causes of different light levels between the eyes; but a large enough group of such cells can – another example of population coding. A shift in the image of only a few thousandths of a millimetre (the smallest parallax we can detect) changes the amount of light in a cone by about 5 per cent, which is enough for single cells to sense. Computer models of parallax detection have simulated the performance of the human observer with complete success.

To discover another advantage of binocular vision, try picking blackberries with one eye closed. We can reach for an object, or thread a needle, more quickly and more accurately with two eyes than with one. As many as 7 per cent of the population fail to develop accurate binocular stereopsis, a common cause being the failure to correct a squint early enough in childhood. These 'stereoblind' people do well enough in everyday life, but laboratory experiments show that they are slightly poorer than controls in one-handed ball-catching and similar tasks. Polyphemus would not have made much of a living from wild berries.

A worse-than-average performance in picking berries may seem a weak argument for linking the evolution of binocular vision to the opposable thumb (which confers upon primates their superior manual dexterity) but evolution by natural selection is the story of small advantages. Take colour vision as an example. We can enjoy the action in *Casablanca* without it. There is nearly always enough information in an image to define an object in black and white, without the need for colour: the object moves; it has shape defined by shading; it has a sharp black–white border – and so on. But the excuse 'it works most of the time' will not help the monkey who has failed to spot the red fruit partly hidden amongst green leaves, amidst dappled light. American engineers sometimes say about a poorly designed piece of apparatus, 'It's good enough for government work'; but 'good enough' is not part of the language of natural selection. Any gene that confers an improvement, however small, will spread amongst the population if its carriers survive to pass on more copies of the gene to the next generation.

Natural selection does not follow the maxim that the best is the enemy of the good. There is always room for improvement.

Texture gradients, familiar size, perspective, motion and binocular parallax: with all these clues to choose from and interpret, our ability to analyse the third dimension rapidly and reliably would seem no more likely than being able to run downstairs whilst reciting *Hamlet* backwards; but this is because we use language to describe the process, as if the visual system were engaged in an elaborate process of reasoning. In fact, 3-D vision is carried out by a number of independent analogue computing circuits, which in the end 'vote' to give us the most likely interpretation. The detection of binocular parallax depends on single cells that have their receptive fields in slightly different positions in the two eyes. The detection of occlusion depends on finding a T-junction, where a line stops at another line, or boundary. Analogue circuits for detecting T-junctions are relatively simple to devise, using the tilted-line detectors discovered by Hubel and Wiesel in the primary visual cortex; and 'T' detectors have indeed been found in parts of the brain (the temporal lobe) devoted to the analysis and recognition of shape.

Another example is 'shape from shading'. Some cells in visual area V4 prefer images where the light source comes from above. If the same image is rotated through 90 degrees, the cells respond less. These cells care less about the position of the blobs in their receptive field than they do about the direction of the shading. Single cells have also been found that respond to texture gradients. They respond to a pattern of dots indicating a surface receding away in depth, but not if the direction of the texture gradient is reversed. Most remarkably of all, these very same cells (in a region of the parietal lobe of the monkey) also respond to surfaces that appear tilted because of binocular disparity. Here is direct evidence that different sources of information about depth are combined by single nerve cells.

There is a final twist in the story of binocular vision. In December 1940 an RAF reconnaissance Spitfire took a stereo photograph while flying high over Cologne. It was an unusually harsh winter in 1940 and the Rhine was full of drifting ice. The story of the 'empty Rhine' was told by the late Babbington-Smith, an Oxford psychologist who was serving in photo-reconnaissance at the time. When the stereo-pair was examined, the observers were bemused to see the ice at the bottom of a deep canyon, rather than floating on the surface of the Rhine. During the time elapsing between the taking of the two photographs, the ice had flowed downstream, giving a false parallax between the two images.

But this explanation of the 'empty Rhine' raises a new problem. How does the observer recognise that a particular piece of ice has floated downstream, when there are so many similar shapes of ice to choose from? Do we have to recognise the exact shape of each piece of ice in order to match it with the same piece in the other eye? This seems implausible, and besides, many of the pieces of ice have a very similar size and shape. The answer to the conundrum of the 'empty Rhine' had to wait until the invention of the 'random-dot stereogram' by Bela Julesz, working in the Bell Laboratories in New Jersey. An example of his invention is shown in figure 4.4. We can think of each picture as a computer-generated ice field, with white dots as ice and black as water. The picture on the right is identical to the one on the left except that the ice in a central square area has moved to the right, giving it a binocular parallax relative to the surrounding ice. When these two pictures are viewed in a stereoscope, the observer sees a central square floating above the background.

Julesz's discovery made it clear for the first time that binocular parallax is sensed *before*, not after, the recognition of objects. The square in the random-dot stereogram is totally invisible in either eye's image alone, and will remain forever hidden to the stereoblind. It exists only by virtue of the relationship between the two eyes. The square is completely camouflaged in the single eye's image, but binocular vision allows us to see it. This idea of camouflage gives us a new evolutionary perspective on binocular vision. A moth might make its colour and texture match that of the bark on which it sits, but it is not able to make itself perfectly flat (although many insects, such as moths and

Figure 4.4 Julesz's random-dot stereogram

Left   Right

butterflies, do their best to be just that). Viewed with two eyes, the moth will leap out from the bark like the square from a random-dot stereogram. This is one reason why birds have excellent binocular vision; and the camouflage-breaking power of stereopsis is exactly what we see when we look upwards through the canopy of a tree. The complexity of the individual leaves and branches destroys the cues to depth seen in *The Five Senses* yet when we open two eyes we can see the trees for the wood.

At first sight camouflage would seem to be especially designed to defeat the parallax sensors in the primary visual cortex. These have receptive fields in slightly different positions in the left and right eyes, so that they are optimally stimulated by a given parallax. However, a random noise field, like a random-dot stereogram, will stimulate nearly all of these sensors – given a white dot in the left eye, there is always either a white or a black dot at a corresponding position in the right eye, and indeed, in every other position. There is nothing special about the central square, except that for every dot in the left eye there is a corresponding dot of the same colour at a fixed distance from it in the right eye. The problem is to discover this fixed distance.

An analogue computer obeys physical laws that parallel those in the outside world. So to solve the random-dot stereogram by an analogue method we must look for the physical laws that describe the relevant aspects of that outside world. One law of optics is obvious and can be used straightaway: if a dot in the outside world projects an image of one colour (black or white) to the left eye, it will project an image of the same colour to the right eye. Therefore we can ignore all the possible matches between black and white dots; the magnitude of the problem has been halved at a stroke. Parallax-sensitive nerve cells do just this: they come in two varieties, one preferring white dots in both eyes, and the other preferring black.

The next bit of physics is more interesting. Random-dot images are difficult to decode because a dot in the left eye has a large number of potential partners in the other eye. If we could reduce the number of individual dots in the image, we would make the problem easier. This can be done by blurring the image. By removing the boundaries between individual dots, blurring replaces individual dots by much larger 'blobs'. Obviously we do not want to go around the world screwing up our eyes to defocus our optics, just to solve random-dot stereograms. The neural analogue computers of parallax do the defocusing for us, entirely in the head. By having large receptive fields, they effectively average the light intensity over regions of the image, and this is exactly what blurring does. The larger the receptive field, the more it blurs the image. By looking at the output of parallax detectors with the largest receptive fields, we can make the solution of the random-dot stereogram easier and easier.

For the final bit of physics we return to Planet Zarg, with its swirling clouds of methane ice crystals. The parallax of each crystal is completely unrelated to that of its neighbour, because all the crystals are at different distances. Luckily, our planet is not like that. The light intensity of neighbouring points in our world is highly correlated; and this is also true of their distance from us. The reason is that our world is made of objects – regions of space where neighbouring points are very similar. The square in the random-dot stereogram is a curious object, because its neighbouring points have no correlation in brightness, but do have a high correlation in distance. This is their Achilles heel for the analogue code-breakers in the brain. To begin with, the random-dot pattern will stimulate a large population of parallax-sensitive nerve cells, including all those for the wrong matches between the two eyes; but suppose that nearby cells in the map talk to one another, as neighbours will. A cell responding to a particular parallax sends a message to similar cells in its neighbourhood (by means of nerve connections), saying: 'Respond more vigorously'. The net result of this is that, if there is an area of the image where the parallax is the same, the cells sensitive to that parallax will win in the competition with the 'wrong' nerve cells.

Computer simulations show that this simple analogue computation solves the random-dot problem particularly efficiently if combined with the other two rules described earlier; but it works only if the nerve cells are laid out in a map, in which neighbours correspond to neighbouring points in the image. Of course, the whole analogue process can be simulated on a digital computer (and indeed this is how it has been tested), but in the real brain it is inconceivable that the cells would be scattered in random locations all over the visual cortex. The problem of wiring the system up during development of the brain would be too great. It is much simpler to have a rule that establishes connections between neighbouring nerve cells. We can predict that there will be maps of binocular parallax, where nearby cells in the map respond to the same parallax. These maps have been elusive, but there is some recent evidence for them in the visual area V5, which contains many parallax-sensitive nerve cells. These seem to be organised into patches where nearby cells have similar parallax preferences, as predicted.

Berkeley equated the perception of depth with the perception of distance, but perception of the third dimension is more complex than he thought. The computation of range is only one of the functions of three-dimensional vision. Distance perception is certainly important for a gibbon leaping between branches, for a chameleon striking at its prey with its long tongue, and for us when we reach out to pick up a cup; but it only part of the story. Shading, texture gradients and parallax do not deliver absolute distances: they tell us instead about the shape of objects, and help us to pick out objects from cluttered backgrounds. There is no single 'range map' in the brain, from which the 3-D world is derived.

The message of 3-D perception is that the brain uses every trick in the book, each one using a specialised analogue computing mechanism. The same is true for the perception of movement, the subject of the next chapter.

5

'Objects moving are not impressed'

The Boulevard du Temple, in Paris, taken by Louis-Jacques Daguerre in 1838 (see figure 5.1), immortalises a blurred shoe-shiner and his patron – the only people who stayed in the same place long enough to register on the film. Daguerrotypes needed exposure times of minutes, rather than the fraction of a second used by modern film. During these long exposures, moving objects were never in the same place long enough to impress their form on the film. Their blurred images are unrecognisable as objects.

Figure 5.1 Daguerre

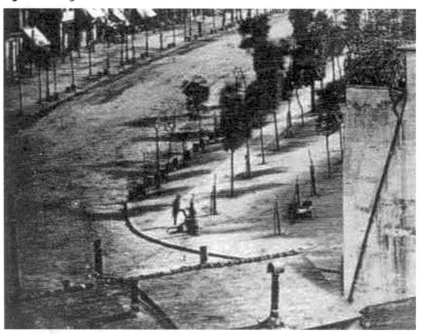

Louis Daguerre sold the rights of his 'daguerreotypes' to the French state for an income of 6000 francs a year for life. His plates were made from silver-plated copper, which he developed in a box containing fumes of iodine. Samuel F. B. Morse, artist and eponymous inventor of the code, was visiting Paris in 1837 and commented on the earliest 'daguerreotypes' in the *New York Observer*:

Objects moving are not impressed. The Boulevard, so constantly filled with the moving throngs of pedestrians and carriages, was perfectly solitary, except for an individual who was having his boots brushed. His feet were compelled, of course, to be stationary for some time, one being on the box of the boot black, and the other on the ground.

At the opposite extreme are modern photographs taken with electronic flash, which can freeze the motion of a bullet, or of a hummingbird in flight. These photographs show us the form of the object, but there is nothing to indicate motion. Indeed, it is difficult for photographers or artists to represent movement accurately. Photographers wishing to communicate the excitement of motion in, say, a horse race, use an exposure sufficiently long to produce motion blur, or they track the moving objects with the camera to produce blur in the stationary background. Cartoonists use multiple images to suggest motion blur (as did the artist Marcel Duchamp in *Nude Descending a Staircase*), or wavy motion streaks behind the moving object. These devices suggest motion, but do not cause the unmistakable sensation of motion itself.

Human vision lies somewhere between the extremes of the daguerreotype and the time-frozen electronic flash. We are not normally conscious of blur in moving objects: nor do we see them frozen in space-time. Instead, we see recognisable objects in motion. Motion is a sensation that cannot be communicated by a single snapshot, but somehow, the sensation of motion can occur without seeing an object in many places at the same time. Motion is a specific sensation, like colour or smell, which cannot be analysed into a series of separate, stationary sensations. Philosophers before Kant failed to distinguish the specific sensation of motion from the events in the physical world giving rise to it, causing much confusion. The most celebrated 'paradoxes' of motion came from the fifth-century (BC) philosopher Zeno of Elea. Zeno's paradoxes of Achilles and the Tortoise, the Stadium and the Row of Solids are neatly summarised in his remark that 'an arrow is where it is'. Zeno's argument was that motion must be an illusion, because the arrow cannot be in two places at once. At any instant of time it must be stationary, so how can it possibly move? In similar vein, the paradox of Achilles and the Tortoise imagines Achilles giving a head start to the tortoise and then setting off to catch up. Say that Achilles takes 1 second to reach the tortoise's starting position. In the meantime the tortoise has moved on, and Achilles still has ground to make up. By the time he has made up this ground, the tortoise has again moved on, and so on. Achilles has an infinite number of distances to make up before he catches the tortoise, and cannot do so in a finite amount of time. He can never actually overtake the tortoise, however slowly it moves.

Aficionados of the great philosopher de Selby in Flann O'Brien's novel *The Third Policeman* will find an echo of Zeno in the savant's excursion into cinematography. Fresh from his triumph in demonstrating that darkness is due to the accumulation of 'black air', de Selby examines a motion picture frame by frame and finds it 'tedious, containing a strongly repetitive element'. Deducing that motion is an illusion, he invents a machine that causes him to be perceived in certain seaside towns while sitting in his study.

Philosophical paradoxes are conjuring tricks that depend upon distracting the baffled reader's attention at the crucial moment. The trick in Achilles and the Tortoise is the claim that an infinite number of distances cannot be traversed in a finite amount of time. This sounds right, but is mathematically incorrect. A finite time interval contains an infinite number of instants, so there is no problem – provided that each of the infinite number of distances is infinitesimally small, which it is. Achilles actually has all the time in the world to catch the tortoise, since even a fraction of the available instants would suffice to run through an infinite number of distances. There is no paradox here. But what about Zeno's argument that motion is impossible, because 'the Arrow is where it is?' How can we see motion without the extremes of blur or a frozen instant?

Victorian popular-science writers had no doubts about the answer. According to the myth that they perpetrated (as we see in the History of Cinematography in London's Museum of the Moving Image [MOMI]), the perception of motion depends upon 'persistence of vision'. Persistence of vision was touted as the explanation of the wonderful new illusion of 'the moving pictures'. The idea was that each frame in a motion picture causes a visual impression that decreases in strength with time. The next frame must follow before the impression of the preceding one decays and this is why motion pictures have to be projected rapidly to be satisfactory. A plethora of parlour toys – the zootrope, the phenakistoscope and others – illustrated the principle. The phenakistoscope has two images of a motion sequence on opposite sides of a card, which is rotated rapidly to give the impression of a parrot leaping in and out of its cage. An anonymous writer in the *Popular Educator* of *circa* 1870 tells us that these toys were hugely popular:

> The enormous sale of these toys reminds the historian of optical toys that the like success attended the sale of Sir David Brewster's kaleidoscope; indeed the popularity of both contrivances brings home to us the truth of Goldsmith's words – 'And still they gazed and still their wonder grew.' And deservedly so, for both have become regular inmates of the toy cupboard ... There are, however, optical contrivances which take a high position on account of the very ingenious manner in which they are contrived; and amongst machines that illustrate the various phases of 'persistence of vision' none are more interesting than those invented by Mr. John Beale, of Greenwich – invented not for any personal advantage, but for the advancement of scientific recreation.

Alas for Mr Beale, who had no thought of personal advantage but only for the advancement of scientific recreation: he would find no place in the modern scientific university. His 'automatic picture' showed the face of a charming young lady, who, waking from an apparent lethargy, rolls her eyes, opens and shuts her mouth, and occasionally, for the special delectation of 'rude boys', pops out her tongue, or varies the amusement by grinning horribly.

'Persistence of vision' undoubtedly exists, and is best seen in the dark-adapted eye; but it is not a sufficient explanation for the perception of motion. An early description of persistence is found in Leonardo's notes on Optics: 'For if when the eye is fixed you draw a brand of fire in a circle or from below the eye upward this brand will seem to be a line of fire which rises upwards from below, and yet this brand cannot actually be in more than one part of this line at any one time.' Leonardo also remarks that stars form circles of fire when the eyes are unsteady. We see these circles when looking at stars through binoculars, unless the hands are held extremely still. Newton, in his *Optics*, also describes the circles of fire that are seen when a brazier of burning coals is whirled around the head (what the Bursar of Trinity College thought about these hazardous experiments is not recorded). Firework displays rely for their effectiveness upon persistence of vision. The dramatic rosettes produced in the sky by an exploding rocket would be disappointing in a one-thousandth-of-a-second exposure on a camera film: we should see only a galaxy of points of light. It is the persistence of these moving points in our vision that produces the pattern.

In all these cases, though, persistence of vision *replaces* the sensation of motion. The dark-adapted eye is poor at seeing fast motion, while the light-adapted eye is poor at persistence of vision. A firework whirled around the head is a poor spectacle in daytime, but at night (when we are dark-adapted) we can use it to write our name in the air. The function of persistence in the dark-adapted eye is to compensate for low light levels by adding the photons up over time, producing a strong signal, but one that is smeared over time (like Daguerre's photograph of the Boulevard du Temple). The same thing happens in night-vision binoculars. They amplify the signal to its limit, and suffer from obvious motion smear. Smear has become the cinematographic cliché for indicating night vision, just as the dumb-bell vignette is the cliché for binoculars.

Persistence of vision is not a sufficient explanation of motion. The true account of motion perception was first put forward by the nineteenth-century German physiologist Sigmund Exner, who argued that motion is a unique sensory experience, produced by a specific brain circuit, rather than a deduction from a temporal series of distinct sense impressions. Exner was a polymath. As well as solving the mystery of motion perception, he was fascinated by sound recording, and founded the Phonogramm-Archiv in Vienna, where early recordings of Bushmen songs can still be heard. He observed the apparently effortless soaring behaviour of buzzards on one of his walks in the mountains and carried out experiments described in his paper 'On the Floating of Birds of Prey'. He produced the first photograph taken through the eye of an insect.

In his experiments on motion perception, Exner first reduced movement to its bare essentials. He flashed an electric spark in one position, followed a few thousands of a second later by a second spark in a nearby position. The observer saw a single spark apparently moving between the two positions. Exner then decreased the spatial gap between the two positions until the jump was so tiny that the motion was only barely visible. He found that he could still see motion when the spatial jump was as little as 2 arc seconds of angle in the eye (the equivalent of the thickness of a sheet of ordinary writing paper viewed from several metres, or a distance on the retina of one sixth of a micron). If two sparks are presented *simultaneously* at this tiny spatial separation, they are seen not as two but as one – like the double star Mizar in the tail of the Plough, they are too close to be distinguished. It follows that 'persistence of vision' would simply cause the two sparks to appear as one, rather than as a spark moving from one place to another. Similarly, if two sparks are presented in the same position a few thousandths of a second apart, we cannot tell whether there are two or one, so it cannot be perceived temporal order that gives us the sensation of motion.

Exner described a simple neural circuit that could compute the direction of motion – the 'coincidence detector'. A moving object first stimulates a receptor in one position on the retina, and then, after a short delay, a receptor some distance away. The signals from the two receptors are sent to a nerve cell, which fires only if the two signals arrive simultaneously. To ensure that this happens, the signal from the first position is delayed by another nerve cell – or a synapse – for the time that it takes the object to move from the first position to the second.

This means that our 'coincidence detector' will fire if the object moves in the correct direction, but not if it moves in the opposite direction. (If it moves from right to left, the second signal is delayed and the messages from the two positions arrive one after the other.) We have a *directionally sensitive* mechanism, which can discriminate the direction of motion. 'Persistence of vision' cannot explain directional sensitivity. If all the images of a moving horse in a movie persisted, we would not know in which direction it was running.

The problem with Zeno's paradoxes of motion is now clear: Zeno invites us to consider motion as a series of frozen space-time images, and then proclaims that motion is impossible. The answer is that we never see the frozen series at all. We should not confuse the sensation of motion with physical motion, whatever that might be. At the fundamental level of physics, motion may not be continuous; after all, electrons jump from orbit to orbit within the atom without traversing intermediate positions, since their quantum states are discrete. Physical time may consist of steps, like the movement of the second hand on a watch. There is no point trying to reconcile these claims with our sensation of motion. Motion is a specific sensation from a particular class of neural mechanism, just as colour is a sensation. We cannot

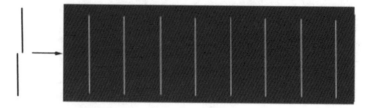

Figure 5.2 Vernier-slit experiment

divide sensation of motion into separate pictures like the frames of a motion picture, because those sensations were never there to start with. Motion is computed directly from the image, without sensory intermediates.

A simple experiment to show that motion is not perceived as a series of frames is shown in figure 5.2. We take a piece of black card with a series of narrow slits cut in it, and behind these slits we move a second card on which a pair of staggered black lines is drawn. As each line passes behind a slit it becomes visible for a brief instant, and if the movement is fast enough, we see a line that moves from slit to slit. This is in fact just a simple Victorian toy for producing a motion picture, called (for no obvious reason) an anorthoscope. Since the lower line is displaced to the left, we see a moving pair of lines, with the lower one displaced to the left. This may seem obvious, but if we follow Zeno or de Selby in examining the movie frame by frame, we shall find, not only that they have a 'tedious and repetitive element', but that the bars are never present simultaneously. Even if we compare their most-nearly simultaneous presentations, they too are in perfect alignment. If, as Zeno would have it, 'a bar is where it is', we should see the bars as aligned. Instead, we see the delayed bar as *lagging all the time*. Even if the lower bar appears in each slit one thousandth of a second later than the upper bar, observers see it as spatially offset. The lag in time between the two bars is indistinguishable from a misalignment in space. No wonder, then, that the German physiologist von Pulfrich, considering the problem of motion, was moved to quote from Parsifal: '*Du sieh'st, mein Sohn, zum Raum wird hier die Zeit.*' ('See, my son, how Time is changed here into Space.' Pulfrich's effect is described in the Appendix, on 'Demonstrations'.)

Victorians called moving pictures an illusion, and projected them in the same theatres where illusionists (magicians) held sway. However, the term 'illusion' requires very careful handling. It is pointless to define an illusory perception as one in which we see something other than the physical reality outside us: we have no idea of what physical reality should look like, apart from our perception of it, so this definition gets us exactly nowhere. A slightly more sophisticated idea is that an illusion causes us to make a mistake, which we would be forced to admit when given further evidence – as, for example, when we see the 'harvest moon' as larger than the Moon at its zenith. Even this definition raises problems, but if we accept it for the moment and apply it to the moving-slit experiment, there is no illusion. We perceived two lines with a gap between them moving continuously behind a series of slits. Isn't this exactly what occurred, and if so, where is the illusion? Of course, if we examined what happened in the image at the back of the eye, we would find no movement – only a succession of stationary flashes; but to deduce from this that we have experienced an illusion is to suppose that there are other occasions when we see what is on our retina correctly. There are no such occasions, any more than there are special occasions when we really and truly see what is 'out there'. The best we can hope for from perception is that we see what is 'out there' well enough to avoid unpleasant surprises; and if we were shown a stationary pattern that we had previously seen moving behind the slit, we would not be at all surprised, because it would correspond pretty well to what we had seen when it was moving.

The same is true of the ordinary motion picture. The camera takes pictures at 24 frames per second, and later on, the film is projected with several exposures for each frame so that the rate of flicker is too high to be perceived. The rate of 28 frames a second is fast enough to represent most movements faithfully, so there is no illusion here. Only if the movement is repetitive and faster than the frame rate do we start to see illusions. If the movement is too fast, it will be 'undersampled' and may seem to be reversed, like the wagon wheels in classic westerns. Michael Faraday observed this effect when looking through roadside railings, and made 'Faraday's wheel' to demonstrate it.

So much for the theory of 'coincidence detectors'. Do they actually exist in the brain? The first to be found were in the retina of the rabbit, where they have the function of warning the animal as quickly as possible of the approach of a predator. These detectors fire vigorously to the image of an object crossing the retina in their 'preferred direction', say left to right, but not to an object moving in the opposite direction. Insects like bees and the housefly also have motion detectors in their eyes. Primates like ourselves do not have motion detectors in the retina, but they were found in the primary visual cortex of monkeys by Hubel and Wiesel. These 'directionally selective' nerve cells responded vigorously to a bar moving in one direction across their receptive field but not to a bar moving in the opposite direction.

Exner's coincidence detectors have some surprising effects on our perception of motion. One is the 'reversed motion phenomenon' (see plate section). If we have a simple two-frame movie and reverse the contrast of the second frame into its photographic negative, the movement appears reversed. For example, if we see a movie of a parrot in its cage fading into the photographic negative of the parrot out of its cage, the bird appears to leap into its cage, not out of it. Computer simulations of 'coincidence detectors' show the same effect. The coincidence detector, being a simple-minded device, does not respond to objects but to the movement of light across its receptors. When a bright spot moves from left to right, light moves across the detector from left to right; but if the spot moves and changes to black, the net movement of light over time and space is in the opposite direction. 'Reverse phi', as it is called, would never have been predicted by Zeno or de Selby, examining their movies frame by frame for the movement of objects.

Our simple-minded mechanisms are also fooled by the 'waterfall effect'. Historical reports of this phenomenon reflect national temperament. In the Austro-Hungarian Empire it was observed after inspecting endless columns of marching troops. In Goethe's Weimar it was noted after prolonged contemplation of a river from a bridge, probably while thinking about suicide. In Scotland it involved a walk in the rain. The Edinburgh solicitor Addams described his observations on the Falls of Foyers in the *Proceedings of the Royal Society of Edinburgh*, in 1834. Addams observed the falls for a while and then noticed, on transferring his gaze to a rock face, that it seemed to move in the *opposite* direction to the water. The same effect is seen in the rolling credits after a TV programme or film: when the credits stop, the screen seems to move in the opposite direction.

The waterfall effect is similar to seeing complementary colours after staring at a saturated coloured patch. If we stare for a few minutes at a saturated red and then transfer our gaze to a yellow, we see the latter tinged with green – the complementary colour of red (see plate section). Similarly, if we stare at a curved line, a straight line will appear curved in the opposite direction; and so on. The explanation of complementary after-effects is to be found in a trick that the brain uses over and over again to improve the reliability of its sensory signals – a trick that was illustrated in horrific circumstances by the night-bombing of Coventry by the Luftwaffe on the night of 14–15 November 1940.

As related by R. V. Jones, then a twenty-eight-year-old junior member of Scientific Intelligence, the raid was carried out with surprising accuracy, at a time when British aircrews were having difficulty in finding Germany reliably at night, let alone a particular city. Scientists knew that the Luftwaffe navigators were following a radio beam emanating from a beacon located in France, but this by itself would have not have given sufficient accuracy, since a radio beam spreads out more and more widely the further it is from its source. Flying down the centre of the radio beam is difficult, because the beam spreads out and becomes weaker as it travels from the source, making it impossible to tell from the strength of the signal whether one is a long way away, or off to one side of the beam. For practical purposes, then, a single beam is useless. The 'Lorenz beam' solved this problem by having *two* radio antennae transmitting dots and dashes alternately, along two overlapping beams. When the dots and dashes fused into a single tone, the navigator knew that he was on a line leading directly to the target.

Motion detectors use a similar method. Nerve cells in the retina and the rest of the brain are never completely silent but have a random level of firing referred to in engineering jargon as 'noise'. ('Noise' means any random event, not just an auditory nuisance.) Noise arriving simultaneously at the coincidence detector from its two inputs will be interpreted as a motion signal, giving a visual equivalent of tinnitus. It is no use ruling out weak signals, because this would also rule out motion signals arriving from real signals of low strength. The solution is to introduce a second detector. A detector of leftwards movement is paired with a rightwards detector. If the two detectors are firing nearly equally, there is probably no external motion signal. If the leftwards detector fires more strongly than the rightwards detector, then the motion is leftwards, and vice versa. By comparing the outputs of two detectors, tuned to opposite directions of motion, a more reliable signal can be obtained.

The snag is that prolonged stimulation of any neural mechanism decreases its sensitivity. A nerve cell given a strong stimulus starts out firing enthusiastically, but soon loses interest and reduces its response to a fraction of the starting value. When we look at the waterfall, the 'downwards' detectors become fatigued and decrease their firing rate. (This is why we habituate so rapidly to speed on the motorway.) When we look at a stationary stimulus, which would normally stimulate upwards and downwards detectors equally, the fatigued 'downwards' detectors fire less than the virginal 'upwards' detectors. The resulting imbalance causes us to see upwards motion.

Movement on the retina has two possible causes: movement in the outside world, and movement of our own bodies. Telling the two apart is important for survival. Motion of the image on the retina is just as important for keeping our balance as for attracting our attention to a moving insect. (Try to stand on tiptoe with arms outstretched and eyes closed!) The main difference between movement of the fly and movement of the body is that the latter causes movement of the whole retinal image. When we move forwards, the retinal image expands from the point we are looking directly at. This principle of 'optic flow' is used in computer games to give the impression of rapid locomotion towards a goal. The goal itself, provided we are looking at it, seems stationary, but all the objects around it move away from it, slowly at first, and with increasing rapidity as they flow outwards. The importance of optic flow was first recognised by psychologists studying the vision of pilots in 1941. At the time it was widely believed by the experts that accurate judgement of distances was essential for landing. Volunteers with less than 20/20 vision in both eyes were judged not to be able to see distance sufficiently accurately, and stood no chance of becoming pilots. The psychologist 'C' Grindley flew in a training aircraft with instructor Peter May and received a quite different account of the way to land: 'You look at the point where you want to land and fly towards it until the ground explodes around it . . . Then you flatten out.' Grindley worked out the mathematics of this in a secret document numbered FPRC 426 and entitled 'Notes on the perception of movement in relation to the problem of landing an aeroplane' and summarised his theory in a diagram using arrows to represent expansion of the ground away from the landing point.

Single coincidence detectors analyse only a small area of the retinal image and are too small to find the centre of an expanding flow field. To get the big picture, the messages from the local motion detectors must be compared and contrasted. Individual motion detectors can be compared to spies sending their messages to a central intelligence agency, which has the task of putting the different (sometimes conflicting) messages together. Recordings from single nerve cells tell us that the job of putting the big picture together is not done in the primary visual cortex, V1. The cells there all have small receptive fields and respond only to the local direction of motion. However, primary visual cortex V1 sends messages to a variety of 'pre-striate' areas, one of which (named V5 by Semir Zeki) contains nerve cells especially suited to optic-flow computations. Cells in V5 respond to movement over large areas of the visual field, rather than to small local signals. Some of them respond best not to simple movements but to elaborate patterns such as rotation or expansion.

The computation of complex motion fields in V5 and another area called MST explains several illusions of motion – for example, the paradoxical 'rotating wheel' in figure 5.3. When we move the image towards our eyes, keeping our gaze fixed on Exner's nose, the small grating patches seem to rotate like a wheel, the two wheels going in opposite directions. In reality, the patches are only moving inwards and outwards on the retina when we move our head. However, the individual patches are tilted at 45 degrees to their true direction of motion, which means that their movement is signalled most vigorously by detectors in V1, themselves tilted at 45 degrees. These simple-minded detectors signal that all the patches are moving along lines at 45 degrees to the radius of the circle whose centre is the point of gaze. This is exactly what would happen if the patches were both moving out along the radius (expanding) *and* rotating around the circumference. The addition of the two components – expansion and rotation – gives a 45 degree vector, like the familiar example of swimming across a current. Presumably, then, the optic-flow detectors in V5 report both expansion and rotation, which is what we see, although there is no real rotation component.

A neurological patient studied in Munich has damage to the higher centres for motion perception. The patient suffered from a stroke, which appears to have left her primary visual cortex intact, but which has incapacitated areas in the 'motion area' V5. She can see static objects more or less normally but complains of being unable to see motion properly. Traffic is a particular hazard, since she cannot tell whether approaching cars are likely to hit her if she crosses the road. She is very poor at judging velocity. In other words, while the normal observer can tell readily whether a car is approaching too rapidly to be avoided, this patient cannot. It would be an exaggeration to say that she sees only a stationary world, but she is unable to use motion perception for the main purposes that make it so valuable.

Motion perception depends on specialised mechanisms in the brain, as does cyclopean vision. Naturally, they are related. Motion parallax

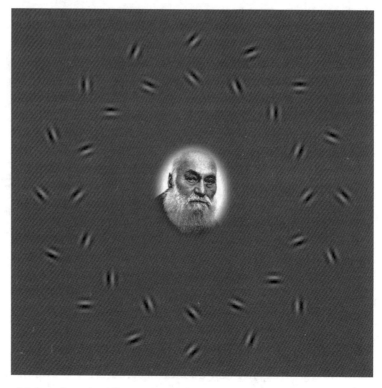

Figure 5.3 Rotating wheel illusion (*Guardian*)

betrays the 3-D layout of the tree when we move our heads. Optic flow tells the pilot when the ground is looming. There is even a special mechanism for responding to differences in motion between the two eyes. If we look at the electronic snowstorm on a badly tuned TV, we see it as flat. However, if we put a sunglass lens over one eye (keeping both eyes open) the noise seems to swirl around in a solid three-dimensional cylinder. The dark lens delays the nerve signals from eye to brain, by increasing the persistence of vision. Strangely, the dimmer eye sees the world later in time than the uncovered eye, by about one-hundredth of a second. (We can get the same effect by really delaying the noise to one eye with an electronic 'delay line'.) The explanation of the 3-D snowstorm is that some of the specialised nerve cells responding to parallax are also directionally sensitive motion detectors. A moving object that stimulates one eye before the other is indistinguishable to these small computers from an object moving in the third dimension.

Motion and 3-D perception tell us the same story about the mechanics of seeing. There are hundreds, if not thousands, of highly specialised mechanisms for analysing the many different kinds of information in the moving image on the retina. When we say that the brain is a 'computer', we should not be deceived into thinking that it is a single computer, like the PC sitting on our desk. Each of the computers making up the brain is a piece of machinery, specialised for carrying out a particular task. 'Computers' like this were known and used long before invention of the PC. The next chapter looks at the history of these analogue computers, from simple machines to predict the tides, to the behemoths that controlled naval guns at the Battle of Jutland.

PART TWO

MAPS AND MODELS

6

'Actual dynamical models of things'

The brain is a computer made of meat, as the AI guru Marvin Minsky said. However, the real question is: 'What sort of computer?' To call the brain a computer is about as useful as saying that a country is a democracy. The old East Germany called itself a democracy, and so does the USA, which wants other countries to be democracies too, so long as they support free-market capitalism and buy McDonald's hamburgers. Democracy is an abstract political theory claiming to give sovereign power to its people; but the interesting question to the people is how this desirable state of affairs is to be brought about, and by what institutions. There are many kinds of computers, as there are many kinds of democracy. To understand how the analogy first came to be made between brain and computer, we have to look back in time before the invention of the PC.

On the eve of VE Day, a young man cycling along King's Parade in Cambridge was thrown into the path of a lorry by a car door opening, and fatally injured. The thirty-year-old psychologist was Kenneth Craik, first Director of the Medical Research Council Unit for Applied Psychology, in Cambridge, and author of the seminal book *The Nature of Explanation*, one of the first to say that the brain is an information-processing computer. Craik's ideas were based on his own experience with computers during the war, and on his experiments with people. When Craik was writing, in 1943, the idea of the brain as an information-processing machine was as new and disturbing as the guidance system on a V2 rocket; now it is confidently assumed in every introductory psychology course.

Until the invention of machines that could perform computations, the activities of the brain had to remain a total mystery. It was compared to a fountain, a telephone exchange, a library or a blancmange – with similarly useful results. A revolution took place when the brain began to be compared with machines that carried out computations. The modern idea that the brain is a machine for processing information is every bit as important as the ideas of Copernicus and Darwin. However, the machines that produced this revolution were not the digital computers of today. They were analogue computers, which solved equations with gear wheels or electrical condensers. Their machinery obeyed an 'analogue' of the equations that they were built to solve. Analogue computers internalised the laws of nature in order to make predictions about the future.

Under 'Computing Machines' in the 1951 edition of the *Encyclopaedia Britannica* the reader is refered to 'Mathematical Instruments'. In common speech at that time, computers were people who did tedious arithmetical calculations, like working out payroll slips. (Female operators, who were the majority, were called 'computeresses' as late as 1960 in England.) The *Britannica* was already out of date on this topic in 1951, but the reference to mathematical instruments reminds us that computers began as measuring instruments, like speedometers and odometers. Unlike modern digital computers, which represent everything in terms of numbers (the French for 'digital' is *numérique*), analogue computers calculate with real moving parts such as wheels and pulleys. An analogue computer is a *model* of some other system, which obeys the same physical laws. Analogue computers can be made out of anything we like, provided they are subject to the same laws as the system they mimic. They can be billiard balls, or even bits of paper. Watson and Crick were using an analogue computer to work out the structure of DNA when they assembled cardboard components representing molecules into a real three dimensional 'model'. The fitting together of the pieces of the jigsaw puzzle in a real spatial framework had to follow laws similar to those of real molecules.

The idea that the brain is an analogue computer was put very clearly by the young German physicist Heinrich Hertz – student of Helmholtz and the discoverer of radio waves – in his *Principles of Dynamics Presented in a New Form*, in 1894: 'The agreement between mind and nature may therefore be likened to the agreement between two systems that are models of one another, and we can even account for the agreement by assuming that the mind is capable of making actual dynamical models of things, and of working with them.'

Hertz was thinking of models like Lord Kelvin's tidal predictor of

1872, preserved in the Science Museum in London. The rise and fall of the tide in any particular place is the result of a number of independent tides, arising from different places. If these tides are 'in phase', they reinforce one another; if they are 'out of phase', they cancel one another out. There are places in the ocean where all the tidal influences cancel out so that there is no rise and fall of tide whatsoever. In 1910 a Dr Whewell predicted such an area eastward of Orfordness and about midway between the coasts of England and Holland. Even earlier, Isaac Newton used the theory of interference to explain the baffling tides in the Gulf of Tonkin, where there is only one tide a day, and sometimes none. The physicist J. J. Thompson (Lord Kelvin) wished to avoid the tedious and repetitive computations involved in calculating the sum of several tides with pencil and paper. His tide predictor was based on the simple principle that a point on the circumference of a rotating wheel – say the wheel of a bicycle – changes its height above the ground over time in the same manner as the rise and fall of a single, perfect tide. The rise and fall is called 'simple harmonic motion'. If we yoke together a number of rotating wheels by strings passing over pulleys, we can add together large numbers of separate 'tidal' influences to move a vertically hanging weight. The movement up and down of the weight represents the rise and fall of the tide. Kelvin's prototype model had eight pulleys; in a later model ten components were added; a 1924 machine in Liverpool could model twenty-six components, and an American machine of 1910 had thirty-seven components which could calculate tidal curves for seven years in just 12 hours.

Lord Kelvin used a computer to predict the movement of water, but we can just as easily reverse the process and use water as a computer. Another analogue computer in the Science Museum was the brainchild of New Zealand born Bill Phillips of the London School of Economics (see plate section). His computer represented the flow of money around the economy by the movement of coloured liquid around perspex pipes. The operator could simulate the effects of tax rises or spending increases by opening and closing valves. One copy even found its way to the Bank of Guatemala, where occasional mishaps flooded the floor with liquid cash.

A model can be a physical structure, like a tide predictor or a 'model' aeroplane in a wind tunnel; but it can also be a mental construction that we use to help us to understand the world. Hertz put these two senses of the word 'model' together when he said that 'the mind is capable of making actual dynamical models of things, and of working with them'. These 'actual dynamical models of things' are the same as our mental models – in other words, the same as our consciousness of the outside world.

'Prediction is very difficult,' said physicist Niels Bohr, 'especially if it's about the future.' Naval gunnery is a good example. In the early days of naval warfare, aiming and firing guns was not difficult. Nelson's gunners at the Battle of Aboukir Bay, in 1798, had no calculations to perform; their battle was won with brutally unsophisticated weapons throwing the maximum weight of metal at point-blank range. ('Point blank' means that no correction for distance is made when pointing the gun.) Even as late as the American Civil War, the famous naval action between the *Monitor* and the *Merrimac* was fought at 100 yards, and the ships were to all intents and purposes not moving. However, by the Second World War, distances and speeds had increased dramatically. The battle cruiser *Hood* was sunk on 24 May 1941, in the Battle of the Denmark Strait by a single plunging shell from the German pocket battleship *Bismarck* fired at a range of range 7.2 nautical miles (13.3 km). A gigantic explosion blew the ship apart. Out of her crew of 1418 men only three, Midshipman William Dundas, Able Seaman Robert Tilburn and Signalman Ted Briggs remained. The first, and a subsequent, Board of Enquiry concluded that a shell from *Bismarck* had penetrated the *Hood*'s comparatively light deck armour (she was a battle cruiser, not a battleship) and detonated the aft magazine. The recent discovery and investigation of the wreck of *Hood* have not altered this conclusion.

Bismarck needed a complicated model to hit such a distant and fast-moving target as *Hood*. First, the range, speed and bearing of the target had to be measured, but this was just the beginning. The firing ship is pitching and rolling, so the gun has to be fired at exactly the right moment. Between the time the shell is fired and the time it lands, the target ship will have moved. The time of flight of a British 13.5 inch gun for 20,000 yards' range was 34.7 seconds. *Hood* and *Bismarck* both had top speeds of about 30 knots, so they could change relative position by 0.5 nautical miles during this time. The shell must be fired at the future position of the target, not at its present position. Future position is particularly hard to calculate if one of the ships is turning at the time. 'The model' must also include the effect of wind on the shell during flight, determined by wind strength/direction and time of flight; lateral drift of shell due to rotation during flight (caused by rifled gun barrels); and minor effects, such as atmospheric pressure and barrel erosion due to previous firings, which affect initial velocity and thus flight time.

In 1898 Captain Percy Scott, RN invented the 'continuous aim' system of gunlaying to deal with the problem of yaw and roll. Before Scott's invention, guns were fired at the top of the roll, when the ship was momentarily stationary. 'Firing on the roll', as it was called, required the gunner to begin his firing movement just before the top of roll, to compensate for the inevitable time-lag between starting the movement, and the gun actually firing. In other words, the gunner had to compensate for his own reaction time. Astronomers already knew how difficult this was. They timed the moment at which a star crossed the meridian by listening to a ticking clock, estimating, for example, that the transit took place at two-thirds of the interval between the fifth and sixth tick. Each observer had his own 'personal equation' for correcting his reaction time – hard enough in a comfortable observatory on dry land, but next to impossible for gunners in the heat of battle.

To overcome the problem of reaction time, Percy Scott removed the sights from the gun and replaced them with a telescopic sight indirectly linked to the movement of the barrel. The indirect mechanical linkage followed the movements of the gun barrel but eliminated the recoil. The gunner looked continuously through this sight, turning wheels to keep the target in the centre, and these same wheels moved the gun barrel rapidly through a system of gears. Improvements over the old system of 'firing on the roll' were spectacular. In 1899 the 4.6 inch guns of the cruiser *Scylla* made fifty-six hits out of seventy shots during the annual prize firing, six times better than her performance the previous year without 'continuous aim'.

Evolution of the eye and brain had anticipated Percy Scott's system. The brain has a continuous aim system for stabilising the eyes when the head is moved, which explains why we continue to see clearly when jogging or playing tennis. Signals from the organs of balance in the inner ear keep the image of the world stable on the retina by moving the eyes automatically in the opposite direction to the head. The vestibulo-ocular reflex, as it is called, is the reason we can still read a book while shaking the head from side to side, or nodding it up and down. However, if we move the book instead of the head, the letters are too blurred to read. (Like most psychological experiments, this is best done in private.) Movement of the book is not detected by the ear, so the vestibulo-ocular reflex fails.

Natural selection did not anticipate the motor car, and trying to read in a car on a winding road fools the eye–ear reflex completely. The reflex tries to compensate for the signals coming from the ear, but the book and the head are actually moving together, so these compensatory movements succeed only in moving the image of the book on the eye. The brain signals its displeasure by making us want to vomit, perhaps because failure of the vestibulo-ocular reflex is usually an early-warning sign that we have been poisoned (as in the case of alcohol). Some antibiotics destroy the reflex also, and before this was discovered, doctors inadvertently produced many patients who experienced an unstable visual world when they moved their heads.

The success of the vestibulo-ocular reflex depends on a very fast direct pathway from ear to eye. But Percy Scott's gunners were turning wheels rather than moving their eyes, so how did they react quickly enough to keep the target in the centre of the sight? Suppose that the gunlayer has the target in his sights, and his own ship rolls to starboard. The target leaves the centre of the sights in the image on the retina and this will be registered some time later by the visual cortex of the gunlayer, who now plans the movement needed to bring the target back to centre. A further delay ensues while the messages are sent from the brain to muscles and finally the adjustment is made. By this time the roll and yaw have continued, or even reversed, and a new correction is needed. It would seem that the gunlayer is doomed always to be lagging behind the movement of the ship, with his gun pointing in the wrong direction.

The gunner must learn to *anticipate* the roll, rather than merely reacting to it. Some forty years later Kenneth Craik realised that observers could use prediction as well as 'feedback' and studied the phenomenon in the laboratory. Observers used a pen to track a rapidly moving object. Provided the movement was regular and predictable (for example, if it was like the movement of the tides in Kelvin's machine), observers soon learned to follow the movement of a target with no reaction time. They formed an internal model of the moving object in their minds. Craik and others used the principle of an internal model in designing predictive anti-aircraft guns for shooting down V1 'doodle-bugs' before they reached London.

This is presumably how Percy Scott's gunners learned the system of continuous aim. Unlike gunners using a 'personal equation' to 'fire on the roll', they would have received continuous updating of their internal model from the position of the target in the sight; but the fire-control problem is still far from solved. The gun must send the shell to the future position of the target, not its present position. To solve this problem, the inventor Arthur Pollen developed his 'Aim Correction' (AC) system, based on an analogue computer. Since the term 'computer' had still to be invented in the 1914–18 war, the machine was quaintly called a 'clock' – the Argo clock.

Arthur Pollen had an unusual background for an inventor. His father, John Hungerford Pollen, was a follower of Cardinal Newman's Tractarian Movement in Oxford, and his son's early interest was in literature rather than science. However, in 1898 Arthur Pollen became (through marriage) Managing Director of the Linotype Company, then depending on some of the most advanced machinery of the time. There is a parallel here with his American counterpart in fire-control systems, Hannibal Choate Ford, who worked for a while at the Crandall Typewriter Company, Groton, NY. On a visit to Malta in 1900 Pollen happened to see a gunnery exercise where two ships fired at a towed target at a range of 1500 yards. He was aware that naval guns had a much greater range than this and asked his naval companions why greater distances were not used. They replied that accuracy at greater distances was impossible, partly because long-distance rangefinders were not available. This began a lifelong obsession for Pollen, in which he tried first to develop – and then, unsuccessfully, to sell to the Admiralty – integrated systems of rangefinders and 'Aim Correction' to solve the fire-control problem.

The Navy already used several clever analogue devices in fire control, especially an instrument invented in 1902 by Lieutenant John Dumaresq; set with the courses and speeds of the firing ship and the target, and the target bearing, the device calculated the rate at which the range was changing, and the deflection of the gun in the horizontal plane. The 'dumaresq' has a complete analogue model of the whole problem, including a little model of the target, which was adjusted in size to represent its speed. Elevation now had to be calculated from range (given by the rangefinder) and the rate by which the range was changing. In mathematical terms, the rate signal had to be integrated, and this was done by the Vickers 'clock', which ran at a rate proportional to the rate change, and which indicated target range on a dial from moment to moment. There were no direct connections between rangefinders, the dumaresq and the Vickers clock, so a considerable amount of work still had to be done by hand. Arthur Pollen

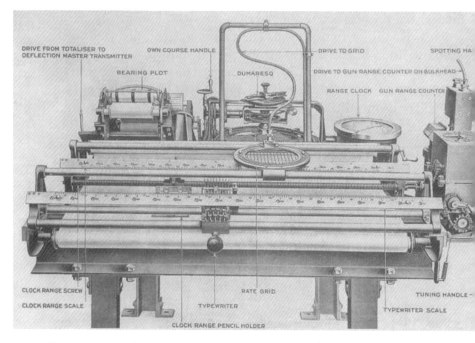

Figure 6.1 An analogue computer: the Dreyer Table Mark 1

set himself the task of designing an automatic system: the Argo clock, Mark II.

The reasons why the Admiralty finally decided not to adopt the Argo clock are still surrounded in controversy. They adopted instead a rival system by Frederic Dreyer – the same Admiral Sir Frederic Charles Dreyer who by an irony hoisted his flag on HMS *Hood* in 1927. The 'Dreyer table' (see figure 6.1) was less automatic than the Argo clock, and there have been persistent suggestions that the Navy adopted an inferior instrument because Dreyer was an insider. The Dreyer table was tested in the First World War at the Battle of Jutland, where the British Grand Fleet was commanded by Admiral Jellicoe, who (according to First Lord Winston Churchill) 'was the only man on either side who could lose the war in an afternoon'. He did not lose the war, but he did suffer heavy losses, the causes of which have been hotly disputed. In a curious book, *The Great Naval Gunnery Scandal*, Arthur Pollen's son argued that that the disappointing performance at Jutland, particularly of Beatty's Battle Cruiser Squadron, was a direct result of the inferior Dreyer table. According to the distinguished naval historian Jon Tetsuro Sumida in his book *In Defence of Naval Supremacy*, Pollen was shabbily treated and the decision to use Dreyer's table rather than the Argo clock was a mistake; but the matter remains controversial. In a recent thesis, 'Fire control for British Dreadnoughts', John Brooks argues that Beatty's tactics rather than Dreyer's tables were responsible for his losses. Not even Beatty blamed fire control for his losses at the time. His much-quoted remark (just after the *Queen Mary* blew up): 'There's something wrong with our bloody ships today, Chatfield,' probably refered to his ships' inability to take hits rather than to their gunnery performance. After all, as Brooks points out, the German fire-control systems at the time were no more advanced than the Dreyer table.

Mechanical analogue computers reigned supreme for fire control up to the end of the Second World War, and the term 'computer' began to creep in to describe them, notably in Hannibal Ford's 'Computer Mark 1'; but by the end of Hitler's war the writing was already on the wall. The first step was to replace mechanical moving parts with electrical components such as condensers, to carry out integration and other mathematical calculations. The process had begun earlier in the First World War, but was resisted by serving officers, who preferred computers they could fix with a screwdriver if they went wrong. (We may sympathise when fuming at the end of a so-called 'computer helpline'.) The final death of the analogue computer seemed to be heralded by the arrival of the stored-program digital computer, first developed for code-breaking. Instead of solving equations by internal mechanical models, the digital computer could solve equations numerically, making the analogue computer an anachronism. But even while this was happening, analogue computers were preparing a secret comeback, in the innocent form of 'switching networks' – now known as 'neural networks'. The story of switching networks begins in the 1890s, in Kansas City.

Almon B. Strowger was an undertaker with a problem. Callers who asked to be connected to Strowger found themselves mysteriously connected to his competitor instead – by the competitor's wife, who ran the local telephone exchange. Strowger was sufficiently incensed and sufficiently clever to invent the world's first automatic telephone exchange, which opened on 3 November 1892 with about seventy-six subscribers in La Porte, Indiana. The first Strowger telephone would have looked very odd thirty years ago but looks less odd now in the push-button age. Instead of a rotary dial, Strowger's telephone had four buttons that the caller pressed in sequence to indicate the desired number (in fact, since there were fewer than 100 subscribers, only the first two buttons were needed.) The heart of the Strowger exchange was an electrical switch called a 'uniselector', which had a rotating wiper arm and a circle of contacts, with which the arm could make a connection. If the selector moved to position '5', the message would be connected to subscriber number 5 on the exchange. By having a second uniselector on top of the first, two digit numbers such as 56 could be encoded, and so on.

The first person to understand the relation between electronic switching circuits and symbolic logic was the American engineer Claude Elwood Shannon (1916–2001). Shannon was the founding father of the modern information age, defining information rigorously, and measuring the amount of information that could be carried by a communication channel such as a telephone wire (the channel capacity). It speaks volumes about the narrowness of what passes as British culture that the death of this genius in 2001 was hardly noticed by the very communications media that he did so much to make possible. (But then, he was only an engineer, not an intellectual.) Shannon's 1936 master's thesis, 'A Symbolic Analysis of Relay and Switching Circuits', provided the mathematical basis for designing switching circuits using symbolic logic. The two positions of a switch can be called '0' or '1', equivalent in symbolic logic to the 'truth value' of a proposition, '0' meaning 'false' and '1' meaning 'true'. Thus a switching circuit can compute 'true' or 'false' for any input, using rules of symbolic logic. Designing a switching circuit for a particular application becomes simply a matter of finding its equivalent in symbolic logic.

Shannon was interested in biology. His 1941 PhD thesis was on the mathematical theory of genetics, a natural enough subject for the inventor of the first self-correcting code, redundancy and information theory; but the next step of applying switching design and Boolean logic to the brain is associated with two other Americans, Warren S. McCulloch and Walter Pitts. In their eccentrically titled paper 'A logical calculus of the ideas immanent in nervous activity' they compared nerve cells to switching circuits. The basic idea is in the first sentence of their paper: 'Because of the "all or none" character of nervous activity, neural events and the relations between them can be treated by means of propositional logic.' In other words, they proposed treating the 'spikes' of electrical activity generated by nerve cells as 'truth values'. If a spike is present in a certain time interval, the truth value is '1' (true), if it is absent the truth value is '0' (false). This was essentially the same as Shannon's idea for electrical signals in man-made switching

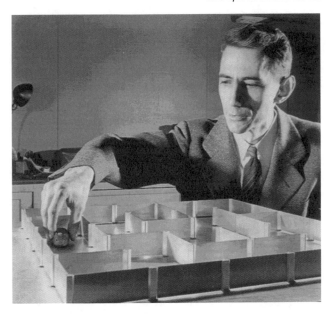

Figure 6.2 Claude Shannon

circuits. The Pitts and McCulloch model is highly idealised and does scant justice to the complexity of the real nervous system. For a start, nerve impulses do not jump directly from one nerve cell to another: they set up chemical reactions at junctions called 'synapses'. When a nerve impulse arrives at a synapse, it starts a complex set of reactions lasting for several thousandths or even hundredths of a second, depending on the kind of synapse. In real nerve cells, it is not clear what it means to say that two impulses arrive 'at the same time'. This timing problem is avoided in the high-speed digital computer by having a very fast clock; to see if two inputs to a transistor are active at the same time, they are consulted only at a 'tick'. The brain, as far as we know, has no master clock of this kind. Another problem is that an incoming spike can activate many thousands of synapses on a single cell, not just a handful as in the Pitts and McCulloch model. The thousands of electrical currents set up on the branching tree of the nerve cell converge and interact in a complex way. Sometimes an incoming nerve impulse will fire the cell, at other times not. Whether a single spike activates the cell is not an 'all or nothing' affair, as Pitts and McCulloch supposed, but is a matter of chance.

Moreover, we now know that the 'strength' of a synapse can be modified by experience. In other words, the probability that a nerve impulse crosses a synapse to activate a cell is in part determined by that cell's history. It is time to leave the idealised world of simple switching circuits, and to enter the more complicated world of machines that learn.

7

Machines that Learn

The problem of learning arose early in the history of switching circuits. Many switching problems are just too difficult to solve by working out the wiring diagram in advance. An example is automatic car number plate recognition, where the input is a TV image of the number plate, and the desired output is a string of letters and numbers. The problem is that some number plates have black numbers, others have white, and all of them vary in brightness depending on the weather and time of day. We would be wasting our time trying to find a letter such as 'B' by looking for a particular value of lightness – say a mid-grey – in the number plate. Even worse, different number plates use different shapes of letters, such as '*B*' and 'B'. A switching circuit to recognise letters seems impossible.

Engineers might never have tried to solve such a difficult problem if not encouraged by the fact that simple brains had solved it first. Even animals without language can be trained to recognise letters. In one experiment, pigeons were rewarded with grain for pecking at a key whenever the letter 'A' in Helvetica typeface was back-projected on to it, and never rewarded when a '2' was present. It was no surprise when they learned to peck only at the 'A'. But the pigeons went beyond this. The first time they were presented with the letter in a new typeface ('Century Schoolbook', for example) they had no hesitation in classifying the letter correctly. They had no problem in dealing with blurred letters, only just recognisable by human observers. They even recognised handwritten 'A's and '2's correctly. The birds had therefore solved a switching problem where the number of inputs could be to all intents and purposes infinite, and the output was 'peck' or 'don't peck'.

Perhaps the pigeons had learned to recognise an 'A' by looking for a simple 'feature', such as a cross-bar in the letter. In fact, the birds were following a much more complicated and initially baffling set of rules. When the pigeons were presented with each of the letters in the alphabet in turn, to see which ones they thought were most like 'A's, the clear winner was the letter 'X', which was pecked almost as much as the original 'A'. The most important feature was having two 'feet' (the pigeons also liked the letter 'H'). But why did they prefer a 'P' to a 'W'? It turned out that the birds were responding not to one feature but to a half-dozen, giving different importance to each of them. This is rather like the decision an experienced punter might make when deciding to back a horse in a race. How well the horse has done in the past is important, but so too are the jockey, the racecourse, the weather, the state of the ground, and dozens of other pieces of information. A successful betting machine would have to take all these factors into account; but it would have to do more. Some factors are more important than others and should be given a higher weight in making the decision. The problem is that even the experienced human punter would have difficulty in telling us what these weights should be. Weights have been learned through long experience, and cannot be put into language. The solution: let the betting machine learn through experience, just as the human punter did, and adjust its own weights. The first machine to do this was called a 'Perceptron'.

The Perceptron was designed by a Frank Rosenblatt, a psychologist working at the Cornell Aeronautical Laboratory. His 1958 paper 'The Perceptron: a probabilistic model for information storage and organisation in the brain' savages the idea that the brain is a Boolean logic computer. The 'all or nothing' principle of the digital computer does not apply to the biological world, where nothing is certain and information is constantly being degraded by 'noise'. Rosenblatt also challenges the idea that memory is a sort of 'trace', or image, of the original input.

> The alternative approach . . . hazards the guess that the images of stimuli may never really be recorded at all, and that the central nervous system simply acts as an intricate switching network, where retention takes the form of new connections or pathways between centres of activity . . . The important feature of this approach is that there is never any simple mapping of the stimulus into memory, according to some code which would permit its later reconstruction. Whatever information is retained must somehow be stored as a *preference for a particular response* (original italics).

In other words, the brain is a highly complicated switching network. For skills like riding a bicycle the theory is obvious. We do not learn to ride a bicycle by forming individual memories of every occasion when we fell off; and if we think about what we are doing, we are distracted and fall off. But it is not nearly so obvious how a switching network could learn to classify letters of the alphabet from 'noisy' images. Here is how the Perceptron does it.

In the Perceptron, as in the Strowger telephone exchange, there are 'input' lines and 'output' lines. In the betting analogy, the input lines correspond to all the factors affecting the performance of all the horses in the race, and the output lines correspond to the horses. Initially, all the inputs are connected to all the outputs. We can imagine each connection as a pipe regulated by a valve. The amount of water flowing through each valve can be regulated. We now need a 'learning rule'. Every time one of the horses wins, the strength of the connections leading to that horse's output unit are increased by a carefully chosen amount. When the horse loses, the connections are weakened.

The devil is in the detail. What is the 'carefully chosen amount' by which the strength of the connection must be adjusted? Remember that every pipe leading into every output unit must be adjusted individually. Several things are obvious right away. If a horse won and was predicted to win, no adjustment is required. If the horse lost and the activity in its output unit was tiny, no adjustment is needed either. If there was no information about the weather in this race, none of the connections leading from the 'weather' input should be adjusted on this occasion. The famous 'delta' rule for learning puts these simple rules into a mathematical equation: each connection is increased or decreased by an amount proportional to the flow of water at its input unit multiplied by the error signal at its output unit.

This much is obvious, and if Bishop Berkeley had proposed a Perceptron he would have stopped right there; but the people who design switching circuits are engineers, not eighteenth-century philosophers. They have to prove that their devices will work, either by building them or by showing mathematically that they will 'do what it says on the tin'. Mathematical proof is better than trial and error, just as it is better to calculate in advance what weight a bridge will bear than to build it and wait to see if it falls down. The high girders of the Tay Bridge would not have blown down if the unfortunate engineer, Sir Thomas Bouch, had calculated the extra load on the track caused by lateral wind pressure on a passing train. The real breakthrough in

Rosenblatt's paper was not the idea of a switching device that learns, which had been proposed many times before, but the mathematics, which proved that it would learn.

A Perceptron-like switching circuit was demonstrated at a 1960 convention of the Institute of Radio Engineers, in New York City, by Bernard Widrow and Marcian Hoff. Widrow and Hoff's 'Adaline' machine (for *Ada*ptive *Line*ar) had a four-by-four array of switches, each of which could be 'on' or 'off'. Their signals were passed through electrical connections to a single summing unit that combined their influences. The operator set the switches into a crude geometric pattern resembling a letter, such as 'T'; and if this was an example of a 'good' pattern then a master switch was set to the 'good' position, otherwise to 'bad'. Inside the machine, 'good' became +1 and 'bad' became –1. Adaline's task was to produce its own output of +1 to 'good' patterns after a period of learning with error signals. The error signal was calculated as the difference between the output of the summing unit and the master switch, and the necessary adjustment was then shared out equally between all the connections.

When a Perceptron learns, it gradually makes fewer and fewer errors. Widrow and Hoff described this graphically as a movement by the machine through an 'error landscape'. Some error landscapes are easily traversed; others are so mazy that the machine never finds its way. A simple error landscape is illustrated by the environment of the swallowtail butterfly, which has a foolproof method for finding a mate. If a swallowtail finds itself on a slope, it climbs it until there is nowhere higher to go. Excelsior! If the landscape has a single peak, all the potential mates and suitors will converge in the lepidopteran singles club. Even if there are several peaks, the strategy will still be a success, because the area on top of the peaks must be less than the area of the landscape as a whole. How do the butterflies find their way upwards? Their vision is too limited to see the distant mountain peaks. All they can do is to look at the landscape immediately around them and decide which direction is the best bet; and the best bet is to go up the slope. The direction of the slope – up or down – can be measured locally. Widrow and Hoff turned the problem of training a neural network into a hill-climbing problem. They imagined a landscape in which every point corresponded to the success of a particular combination of connection strengths in reducing the error. They showed that there was a kind of problem that Adaline could solve merely by copying the swallowtail butterfly. This was because the 'landscape' for this kind of problem had a single peak, and because the best direction to go from any point on the landscape could be calculated directly from the error signal. Contrary to what one might imagine, they proved that the strengths of each connection could be adjusted quite separately, without taking any note of what was happening with the others.

Local hill-climbing will not always work. Imagine the predicament of a butterfly in a field of small boulders, which gently rises towards a particularly high boulder in the middle. Hill-climbing butterflies will most likely come to rest on the nearest small boulder and will never reach the middle. Neural networks are in a similar position if they are in an error landscape with many local peaks. They will hardly ever learn. The solution for the butterfly is to provide frequent puffs of wind that knock it off a small boulder on to the ground. This ensures that it will not dawdle long on any small local bump; eventually it will find the big boulder in the middle. The equivalent of the puffs of wind in neural networks called 'Boltzmann machines' is 'noise' applied to the connection strengths. The noise jiggles the strengths from time to time to stop them complacently staying on a small boulder, and forces them to go hill-climbing again.

When a soap bubble is drawn out between two or more rings, it takes on a complicated shape, very difficult to predict. The shape is not worked out in advance by an omniscient designer, but depends on local interactions between the molecules in the film. The smaller the local curvature of the bubble, the less energy is stored in it. Molecules in a magnetic field and the vortex patterns in fluid flow are other examples of self-organising systems, where apparent intelligence results from purely local interactions. One of the most influential papers in neural network theory was by the physicist John Hopfield, who said that successful neural networks were those that settled – like bubbles – in stable 'least energy' states. These states are similar to the 'minimum error' states achieved by hill-climbing, but Hopfield defined error in such a way as to make it mathematically equivalent to physical energy. The network described by Hopfield evolves over time, like a soap bubble, until it finds an energy minimum. One reason why Hopfield's 1982 paper caused such a stir was his confident statement that 'The model could be readily implemented by integrated circuit software.' This turned out to be true. Only five years later AT&T Bell Laboratories were developing 'neural network chips' based on Hopfield networks.

One day, artificial neural networks could make good the damage to real nervous systems. The brain of a paraplegic patient is intact, but the nerves leading to the limbs have been severed. Somewhere in the brain there must be intact nerve cells that normally fire when we have the intention to move a limb. Why not use the activity of these cells to control a robot limb? Rats have shown the way. Laboratory rodents learned to press on a lever in their cage with the right force and duration to make the robot arm deliver a drink of water into their home cage. While the rat was learning, computers recorded activity from thirty or so nerve cells in a part of the rat's brain (the motor cortex) where cells fire before and during movements. A neural network learned which patterns of firing in the cells best predicted the movement of the robot arm. The output of the network was transformed into a single electrical signal that could itself be used to control the robot arm. In other words, the 'input' into the network was the activity of the thirty or so nerve cells, and the 'output' was an electrical signal to the robot arm (just like an Adaline). When the network had learned, the rat's lever was disconnected from the arm and the signal from the neural network was connected instead. Movement of the robot arm was now controlled by the nerve cells in the rat's motor cortex, via the artificial neural network.

Now the 'neurobiotic' rodents could move the robot merely by thinking about it. Some rats cottoned on to this quickly and stopped bothering to press their lever. This shows that the cells could not be the direct cause of the movements, since they could fire without the movement being made. They are more likely related to the intention to move, the actual movements being organised 'downstream'.

The artificial neural network of the neurobiotic rat learned to predict the movement of the robot arm from the nerve cells in the rat's motor cortex. This notion of prediction can be applied to a classification task, such as recognising a car number plate. An input comes in from a particular letter, say an 'A'. The input is 'noisy' and may be a type of 'A' that has never been seen before. There is no question of saying that this noisy and novel image has *certainly* come from a letter 'A' on the number plate. What we can try to do is to say that the *most likely* letter to have caused this particular image is the letter 'A'. In other words, does the presence of an 'A' in the image do the best job of predicting the noisy image that we have in the input? Here is a new way of thinking about the perceptions of our own brains. Are they informed guesses about the most likely state of the world outside? Are they, indeed 'controlled hallucinations' – controlled by the laws of probability? The next chapter will be about this strange notion, which can be traced to the unlikely source of a mathematical theorem by the eighteenth-century clergyman, the Reverend Thomas Bayes.

8

Controlled Hallucination

'Perception is nothing more than successful hallucination.'
(statement attributed to the AI scientist Max Clowes)

The Reverend Bayes was born in London, like two other founding fathers of computing, Charles Babbage and Alan Turing. His grave is in London's Bunhill Fields, off the City Road, where shoemakers 'popped their weasels' (pawned their tools) to pay for drinks in The Eagle public house. The Fields were a burial pit for plague victims – hence their name, a corruption of 'Bone Hill'. Bayes keeps company in Bunhill with William Blake, John Bunyan and Daniel Defoe. Blake's grave, where he lies with Sophia, is often marked by flowers. Bayes' grave is undistinguished and unnoticed by visitors. Yet Bayes' theorem on probability is now a vital tool for understanding the problem that neural networks and the brain itself have in inferring 'what is out there' from its sensory input. Bayes' theorem assumes that even before collecting any evidence we have a current model of what is out there. The model is called a 'prior' (no ecclesiastical pun intended). After some evidence has been collected, the probability of that model being true has been altered, so a new model is generated called the 'posterior'. In the most abstract possible way, Bayes' theorem describes the kind of computation the brain may be carrying out when we infer the existence of an outside world from our noisy sensory input.

For example, why does a lump of coal look black? The obvious answer is that it casts a dark image on the retina; but the obvious answer is wrong. A lump of coal in bright sunlight reflects *more* light than a piece of white paper under moonlight, yet the coal looks as black in sunlight as it does in a coal cellar. When we perceive coal as black, we are inferring something about the coal itself (its low surface reflectance) rather than perceiving the amount of light reaching the eye. However, surface reflectance is not something that we can know directly: we must infer it from the pattern of light reaching the eye. We must take into account not only the light reflected from the coal, but how much light was falling on it. This is a classical case of Bayesian reasoning. We have to figure out what is the most likely surface reflectance of the object (high or low) given the available information, including prior probabilities, and taking measurement 'noise' into account.

Sometimes our best guess is wrong. The Moon has approximately the same reflectance as a coal tip, but in the night sky it looks brilliant white. Its black surface is illuminated by a giant, invisible spotlight – the Sun. Long before Neil Armstrong set foot on the Moon, psychologists had created a lunar landscape by illuminating pieces of coal with a hidden spotlight in an otherwise dark cellar. The coal glowed as white as the Moon in the night sky. Because we cannot see the Sun or any other objects near the Moon, there is insufficient information available for computing its surface reflectance. The Moon looks white because we have a built-in guess that an object is white if it reflects more light than its surroundings, other things being equal. In the language of Bayes' theorem a guess like this is called a 'prior' – as in *a priori*. The Moon is a white prior.

If the Bayesian philosophy of perception is correct, our perceptions are models, which we use to make informed guesses about the outside world. We are back with Hertz again and his 'actual dynamical models of things'. The process of perception involves selecting an internal model and then checking it against the data. The best model is the one that best fits the data. As Richard Gregory says, perceptions are hypotheses. Sometimes two equally likely hypotheses fit the data, like the ambiguous figures of the duck-rabbit and Necker cube in figure 4.3, and the brain entertains them in turn.

Models of this kind are called 'generative models', because they try to generate the data. This idea has been familiar to statisticians for a long time. A simple example is Kelvin's tidal predictor. The 'model' behind the predictor is that any tide, however complex, can be composed of a set of simple tides, each of them a simple harmonic motion. These components can be called the 'principal components' of the tide. Once we have done a principal components analysis we can invert the process and use the model to produce the specimen tide. In an analogue machine like Kelvin's we could even imagine doing this by producing real oscillations in a water tank. Principal components can be used in many different problems where a simple model underlies complex data. Colour vision is another good example. We know that nearly all natural colours can be distinguished by the human eye using only three types of cone (red, green and blue). This remarkable fact suggests that three components are sufficient to describe natural colour spectra, and a principal components analysis confirms this. Statisticians do component analysis of all sorts of data and then check their model by seeing how well it can generate the data from the model. As it happens, principal component analysis is only one of many kinds of generative model, all of which are related on a deeper mathematical level. Another kind is 'factor analysis', controversially used by Spearman to find the components of human intelligence. Spearman claimed that a particularly simple model fitted the data; nearly all variation in human intelligence was caused by a single variable that he called 'G' (General Intelligence).

Computers use generative models for translating human speech into written words. This is not a trivial task, for there are no gaps in speech corresponding to the gaps between written words. The sensory data – sound pressure waves reaching the microphone or ear – are of little interest in themselves: who cares what the molecules of air are doing in our vicinity, unless we want to avoid a draught? What we really want to know is what the speaker is doing with her vocal cords to *generate* these data. The task is like calculating how many boats there are inside a busy harbour from the ripples and waves outside the mole. Impossible? Suppose we had a model harbour and could move our own boats within it to generate waves and ripples. We could then see which version of the model produced waves and ripples like those coming from the harbour. We might not always get it right, and there might be many different models that produced the same data; but with the right Bayesian priors (no boat is doing more than 5 knots in the busy harbour and no boat is longer than 100 metres) we might get there. Back to speech: we know we have a generative model for sound pressure waves, because we can talk. Run this model backwards and you have a model for interpreting someone else's speech. The idea may seem wild and disturbing; but it works in neural networks. Computers are getting quite good at speech recognition, and as the leading network theorist Geoffrey Hinton puts it: 'All the best speech-recognition programs now work by fitting a probabilistic generative model.'

Generative models are also beginning to explain how we move our muscles. Moving our limbs has much in common with interpreting our retinal images. In both cases the number of possibilities is so vast that we have to simplify them with models. There are roughly 600 muscles in the human body. Even if we assume for simplicity that each muscle can be contracted or relaxed, there are still 2 raised to the power 600 possibilities – more than the number of atoms in the Universe. It does not seem plausible that every possible movement we might wish to make is represented in the brain by a memory of exactly the right signals to be sent to each individual muscle. The alternative is that we in some way represent the desired end state of the movement – an internal model – and have neural networks that we tune by experience to translate these high level models into action. If action involves the comparison between a model and the present state of the body, the distinction between perception and action begins to fade away.

If perceptions are internal models, we should be able to experience them without images on the retina. Dreams and hallucinations tell us that this is so. 'Hypnagogic images' are the dramatic and realistic images that sometimes appear just before sleep. A monotonous day's driving is followed by vivid images of the road, but not the same road as was seen during the day. The images can be bizarre and frightening. People called 'eidetikers' can experience these vivid images even with their eyes open and, in some cases, use them to carry out amazing feats of mental arithmetic on an imaginary blackboard. *The Confessions of an English Opium Eater*, by de Quincy, contains some of the best-known descriptions of drug-induced hallucinations, but de Quincy had a powerful visual imagination even before he followed Coleridge into laudanum dependence. As he put it himself, 'If a man took opium whose talk was of oxen, he would dream about oxen.' Coleridge had been reading about Kubla Khan just before he fell asleep from the effects of an anodyne. De Quincy notes that we can perceive scenes in the shapes of the clouds as well as from opium-generated dreams: 'In the early stage of the malady, the splendours of my dreams were indeed chiefly architectural; and I beheld such pomp of cities and palaces as never yet was beheld by the waking eye, unless in the clouds . . .'

Laughing gas, ether, laudanum and hashish were all regularly and legally used in nineteenth-century 'frolics'. Humphrey Davy, the inventor of the miner's safety lamp, discovered nitrous oxide (laughing gas) and was a confirmed recreational user. After the Napoleonic military adventure in Egypt, returning soldiers introduced hashish into France, where Dr Jacques Moreau tried it out to cure mental illness. When the literary imagination combined with drugs in the Club des Hachichins, the results were predictable: Gautier described '. . . hybrid creations, formless mixtures of men, beasts and utensils; monks with wheels for feet and cauldrons for bellies'. Monks with wheels for feet are quite typical of drug-induced and hypnagogic imagery. Hallucinations combine together normal elements in new ways, but are otherwise conventional. LSD was described by the chemist who synthesised it as producing 'extraordinary plasticity' of form, but the forms are similar to those of normal vision.

Later in his malady de Quincy saw faces everywhere. 'But now that affection that I have called the tyranny of the human face began to unfold itself ... upon the rocking waters of the ocean the human face began to reveal itself; the sea appeared paved with innumerable faces ...' It takes very little in the way of input to hallucinate a human face, as the Man in the Moon testifies. We can see faces in cracks on the wall, in patterned carpets and in stone. The Face in granite (in the plate section) shows a small face selected from hundreds of candidates in the granite paving of Euston Underground Station. Images like these are midway between pure hallucination and normal perception. The face is not entirely invented; it arises from a chance collection of blobs in the image, but these blobs could just as well have suggested something else, such as a bird in flight. As soon as we begin to scan the granite for birds instead of faces, they start to emerge, like developing prints in a photographic darkroom.

Hallucinations tell us that the brain can generate perceptions with minimal support from the retinal image. There is probably very little difference between a drug-induced hallucination and the perception of faces in clouds and random textures. In both case the input consists of semi-random input from the eye. Drugs may scramble the normal input and make it more random, allowing more fanciful interpretations. In the Charles Bonnet syndrome, patients with failing vision start to impose hallucinations on the increasingly meaningless input from their eyes, or perhaps upon spontaneous 'noise' arising directly in their visual cortex. Ordinary perception may bear the same relation to hallucination as memory does to confabulation. Patients with severe memory loss sometimes produce quite detailed 'false memories' to fill in the gaps. They may well experience these memories as real, even though they are invented to cover up the lack of evidence.

The idea of normal perception as 'controlled hallucination' is intriguing, but it raises all sorts of questions. If a perception is an internally generated hallucination that we check against 'data', what are the data? Is it the raw images in the retina, or the messages in the primary visual cortex? What is the nature of the internal model? Is it another kind of image? Is it 2-D or 3-D, coloured or not? And how do we 'check' a model against incoming data? How good must the fit be before we accept it? If a model fails to match the data, how do we set about generating a new one?

Another problem is anatomy. The visual pathway contains specialised analogue computers at every level, without any obvious intervention from an active model. The retina transforms the photons captured by rods and cones into 'contrast' signals in optic nerve fibres. These contrast signals are produced by small analogue computers (retinal ganglion cells) that compare the number of photons captured by neighbouring cones. As far as we know, this process has no need of intervention from a higher-level model. Indeed, the vast majority of optic nerve fibres run in one direction only: from eye to brain, not the reverse. There is no question of checking our internal models directly against the photons absorbed by rods and cones. Only when we get to the thalamus and the primary visual cortex do we begin to find 'feedback' connections running in the reverse direction. In theory, feedback connections would allow us to match upward flowing data with downward flowing hypotheses; but the real function of feedback connections to LGN and V1 remains obscure. The cells in V1 carry out a wide variety of analogue computations on the input, such as determining the local tilt of lines and direction of movement, and there is no compelling evidence that this depends on intervention from 'higher centres'. Some physiologists argue that feedback connections alter the activity of cells at the lower level, but this is hard to believe. The last thing you want in a Bayesian machine is to change the data to fit your theory, like a government that starts to believe its own propaganda.

The retina and primary visual cortex are the wrong places to look for 'hypothesis testing'. Their analogue computers have already been designed by millions of year of natural selection to model the incoming data. A likely compromise between bottom-up and top-down processing is that the image is first analysed automatically by bottom-up processes to put the incoming data into a convenient form for hypothesis testing. Only then does the top-down process of Bayesian inference begin. We shall see exactly this two-stage scenario played out in the recognition of faces, the subject of the next chapter.

9

The Babel Library of Icons

'I never forget a face, but in your case I'll make an exception.'
(Groucho Marx)

In his story 'The Library of Babel', Jorge Luis Borges (who had been director of the National Library of Argentina) describes a library that contains all possible 410-page books. Most of the books are complete gibberish (worse even than *Finnegans Wake*), including one in which the letters 'MCV' are perversely repeated from the first line to the last. Some contain a few lines of obscure dialect embedded in a typographical word salad. It takes the librarians over 100 years to discover that the language of two lines of text in one of the books is a Samoyed-Lithuanian dialect of Guarani, with classical Arabic inflections.

One of the books in the Library of all Books necessarily begins: 'It is a truth universally acknowledged, that a single man in possession of a good fortune, must be in want of a life.' We understand this garbled beginning of *Pride and Prejudice* even though we have certainly never met it before. Most sentences produced by the proverbial monkey on a typewriter would be grammatically illegal, consisting of meaningless words such as 'pxxty', or ungrammatical collections of real words such as 'Please of dog away justice'. Just occasionally, a grammatical sentence might emerge from the chaos, but it would nearly always be fridge-magnet poetry, like 'Colourless green ideas sleep furiously.' Meaningful books in the library are hopelessly outnumbered by gibberish, and the librarians frequently have problems cataloguing them. The same problem arises in the Babel library of images.

As the Babel Library of Books contains all books, the Babel Library of Images contains all images. There are 410 counted images of the Mona Lisa with Mont St Victoire in the background. (Of course, there are many more uncounted.) A puzzling image in the endless ninth gallery of the 40th floor of the north wing is apparently completely random, but according to believers contains the true likeness of God.

Non-believers reply that the image must also logically contain the picture of an elephant. How large is our Library of Icons, and how can we tell which images have meaning? If we followed the example of language, the first task would be to split images into meaningful components like words. The problem is that images are continuous, like sheets of paper lacking spaces and full stops. Luckily we can get round this problem by exploiting the poor acuity of the human visual system. If the image is split into small enough squares or 'pixels' (short for 'picture elements'), we cannot tell it apart from a truly continuous image. Every image can now be represented by a series of numbers, each expressing the amount of light in one pixel. In fact, as the painter Seurat discovered, we can perceive the meaning of an image even if we can see the boundaries between pixels, so the exact choice of pixel size is not that important.

We can now begin to construct a library of images. Like Borges we shall consider 'books' of one size only. Each image will be 256 pixels wide and 256 pixels high, large enough to represent all everyday objects or scenes, including human faces. Each pixel has a number between 1 and 256 representing the amount of light in a small area of the image (we ignore colour for the moment). There will be $256 \times 256 \times 256$ possible books in our library, or about 17 million. Call the language of these books 'Pixelese'. An image of a cup and a section of the same image in Pixelese is shown in figure 9.1.

The vast majority of books in Pixelese will be meaningless, like the example in figure 9.1, where the pixels are filled with random numbers, the visual equivalent of 'noise', like the whispering of a cowry shell held to the ear. Sometimes noise can be confused with a meaningful image. Just by chance, pixels of similar colour can be next to one another and give the impression of a 'blob' or a 'line'. In one of the books in Borges' Library the phrase 'O Time your pyramids' popped out of one book. Was it accidental or did it have a deep meaning? If we add noise to a meaningful image, like the second example in Figure 9.1, the original image is dimly discernible through the fog. This image too will be in our Babel Library. How could the librarians establish that it is meaningful and not just pure noise?

The problem with looking at an image is that we instantly perceive its meaning (if it has one) rather than its pixels. A useful trick for getting round this is to represent an image by a landscape, in which dark regions become valleys and light regions mountain peaks (see figure 9.2). The landscape contains the same amount of information as

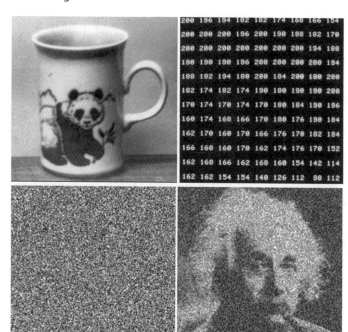

Figure 9.1 Top: A cup and a small section of the same in 'Pixelese'
Bottom: Noise and noise added to a face

the original image, but it might as well be written in a Samoyed-Lithuanian dialect of Guarani. Landscape images tell us that ordinary images are complex physical objects. They contain no obvious structures corresponding to eyes or noses.

Once we get into the habit of thinking about images as landscapes, we can begin to manipulate them. The pictures in figure 9.3 show a face and a blurred version, with their corresponding landscapes. Blurring the image is the same as eroding the landscape. Adding 'noise' to the image as in Fig 9.1 would have the opposite effect to blurring, and would make the landscape more 'spiky'.

All this is discouraging to the librarian trying to catalogue the Babel Library of Icons in Pixelese. Describing even a small image in Pixelese will take over 16,000 'words'. The resulting description will have no obvious meaning. Amongst the 17 million images in the library will be three representing the face of Einstein, his blurred image and his noisy image. Those three will have nothing obvious in common. Very few of their pixels will have the same value. The problem is even

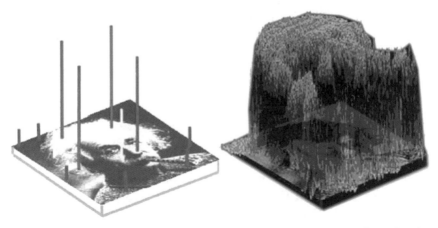

Figure 9.2 Landscapes of faces: how a flat image can be rendered as a three-dimensional landscape. We replace each pixel by a vertical bar, with a height proportional to the brightness of the pixel. The example on the left shows 12 pixels treated in this way. When every pixel is treated, we have the dense landscape shown on the right. Features like Einstein's white hair are now represented as a high mountain range. Note that many of the deep valleys cannot be seen because they are hidden.

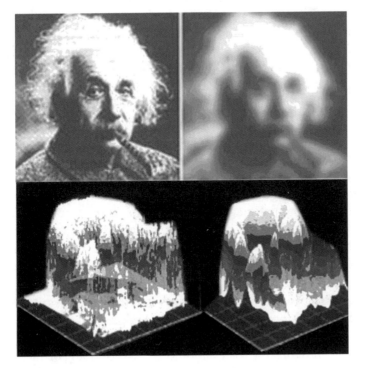

Figure 9.3 Landscapes of a face before and after blurring

worse! There will also be images of Einstein where his face is smaller, or displaced from the centre of the picture. These will have pixel values entirely different from one another. A small change in the lighting of the face will also have a devastating effect on pixel lightness values. Plainly, we are headed in the wrong direction.

If images were random, there would be no alternative to Pixelese. It takes as many words to describe a random image as there are pixels in it, because in a random image the lightness of a pixel cannot be predicted by its neighbours. In a random landscape, one step can take the walker from sea level to the peak of a mountain 20,000 feet high; the next step goes down to 500 feet. You never know what will happen next. But if a landscape has structure, the lightness value of a pixel is more or less predictable from its neighbours, just as in a grammatical English sentence each word is to some extent predictable from the one that went before ('The cat chased the . . .'). Predictable structures in image landscapes correspond to hills, ridges, cliffs and valleys in real landscapes. A 'hill' is a 'blob' in the image, perhaps the part of the image corresponding to the eye of a face. A 'ridge' is a line, along which we encounter similar pixel values. A 'cliff' is a boundary between different regions of the image, for example the horizon between sea and sky.

If images contain these large-scale structures, a pixel-by-pixel description becomes unnecessary, or in grammatical terms 'redundant'. Like the ramblings of a bore, pixel-by-pixel messages say both too much and too little. Ideally, all those boring pixel values should be thrown away and replaced with a précis of the features in the landscape. This is indeed what happens when images are 'compressed'. One of the first images to be sent across the transatlantic telegraph cable was the historic image of Generals Foch and Pershing. So slow was the telegraph that the earliest pictures to be sent across the Atlantic took more than a week to transmit. Engineers soon reduced this time to three hours by exploiting the redundancy of non-random images. A typical trick is 'run-length encoding', which transmits the pixel value of an identical row of pixels once only. 'Image compression' (as it is called) has become a fine art. A familiar example to digital photographers is the JPEG compression standard (the acronym stands for the Joint Photographic Experts Group), which can easily reduce the number of bytes required to transmit an image tenfold without obvious loss of quality. Image compression is the technology that has made pornography possible on the Internet.

The cat in figure 9.4.1 is easily recognised from its abstract outline drawing. Cartoons replace pixels in an image by lines running along

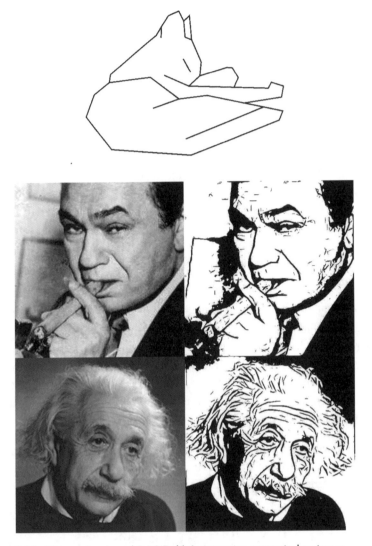

Figures 9.4.1 Attneave's cat, and **9.4.2** Dakin's computer-generated cartoons

ridges and cliffs in the image landscape. Automatic cartoons can be drawn from real images by locating these features (see figure 9.4.2). Many of these features arise from the boundaries that divide the front view of an object from its invisible side. (Think of the Moon, for example.) They are not so much properties of the object itself, but of its projection to the eye. If we miraculously had three-dimensional images of objects in the eye, we should need a four-dimensional space to represent their outline. Cubism was an attempt to deal with this problem, only partially successful. Given that outlines are such peculiar things, it is remarkable that line can convey so much, as the late David Marr pointed out in his book *Vision*. The pixel values of a line drawing are completely different from those of a full image of the object, and yet they can convey to us the same meaning. Marr argued that line drawings are tapping in to a level of representation in our visual system where Pixelese has already been replaced by a 'feature' language. He picturesquely described this early level as the 'primal sketch'. In many ways, the primal sketch is like a line drawing or cartoon.

An early pioneer in using sketches to transmit information across the telegraph was Francis Galton, a cousin of Charles Darwin and the inventor of fingerprinting. Galton's scheme depends on identifying five *cardinal points* – the notch between the brow and the nose, the tip of the nose, the notch between the nose and the upper lip, the parting of the lips and the tip of the chin (see figure 9.5). He devised a code that would put these into four telegraphic 'words', arguing that . . .

> . . . four telegraphic 'words' are sufficient to convey a very fair profile likeness. The cost of sending an extra four words by telegram to any part of the British Isles being only twopence, and of a moderate amount over-seas, the practice of telegraphing profiles of persons of current interest, might become common. A refugee criminal could easily be outstripped by his portrait, sufficiently like him to justify, in connection with corroborative evidence, his being placed for a while under police observation.

Perhaps we recognise line drawings so easily because the brain itself is an artist. A blunder in the History of Optics gave a hint that line drawing begins in the eye itself.

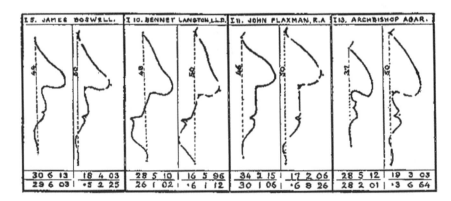

Figure 9.5 Galton's face profiles

The Italian physicist Grimaldi (1613–63) found that light appeared in the shadows of objects where it had no business to be according to Newton's theory that particles of light travel in straight lines. He had demonstrated diffraction. However, diffraction could be explained by the particle theory if particles were deflected when they passed near to an object. The crucial proof of the wave theory of light, later carried out by Sir Thomas Young (appointed Professor of Natural Philosophy in 1801 at the recently founded Royal Institution in London), was the observation of black bands where two light waves cancelled one another out, like the tides in the Gulf of Tonkin. This demonstration eluded Grimaldi. He saw black rings surrounding the fuzzy image of the sun cast through a pinhole; but these were a subjective phenomenon, now called 'Mach bands' after the Austrian physicist who first described them accurately and realised that their cause was in the eye. Ernst Mach made fuzzy boundaries between light and dark areas in an image, and observed strong dark bands just at the point where the dark region started to get lighter. There was a corresponding light band just at the point where the light region started to shade off into dark. These bands represent the first efforts by the brain to substitute lines for pixels. A striking demonstration of Mach bands in a two-dimensional form is seen in a version of Victor Vasarely's 'pyramid' figure (see figure 9.6).

Grimaldi had bad luck with his observations. Thomas Young's black bands could easily have been produced by his eye, but they were not; and his memorial stone in Westminster Abbey tells the happy result. (It says that he 'first established the undulatory theory of light, and first penetrated the obscurity which had veiled for ages the hieroglyphics of Egypt'.) Only in religion is it a sin to be right for the wrong reasons.

Mach proposed a mathematical model for his 'bands'. The retina, he

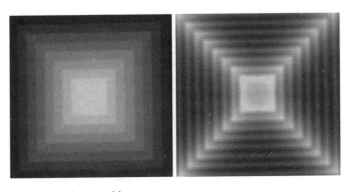

Figure 9.6 The Vasarely pyramid

said, does not transmit the output of individual rods and cones along the optic nerve. Instead, it transmits signals of the *difference* between neighbouring receptors. If this difference signal is positive, a white line is signalled; if it is negative, the band is black. If the difference is zero, no signal is transmitted. The Vasarely pyramid shows how this process produces subjective white lines. An object is seen as black only if it is surrounded by a lighter object or surface. A television picture can show us deep black colours, but as soon as it is switched off, the screen looks grey. The TV set seems miraculously to have subtracted light from its screen; in fact, this phenomenon is entirely subjective, and due to the fact that our retina contains its own contrast control. Mach's inspired guess was eventually confirmed by an unlikely witness – the horseshoe crab. Each fibre from the crab's eye signals the difference between light falling in the centre and in the surround of its 'receptive field'. In effect, the retina replaces the intensity signals in the receptors by a *contrast* signal at places in the image like cliffs and ridges where intensity is changing rapidly. The eye strikes the first blow against the redundancy of Pixelese.

However, we should not get carried away – the retina falls far short of speaking the language of vision. Despite the importance of line, the boundaries of objects are not the only words in the visual lexicon. We do not distinguish between sand and water by their outlines, but by their colour and texture. Texture is what distinguishes the bark of the oak tree from the bark of a beech, or sand from pebbles. It is not the outline shape of each grain of sand that makes a sandy texture, or the individual shapes of leaves and stalks that make a field of wheat.

The brain's description of texture begins in the primary visual cortex. Hubel and Wiesel discovered that receptive fields of single cells in the visual cortex resemble those of the retina in having 'centres' and 'surrounds' that cancel one another out. However, they are not circular like soccer balls, as those in the retina are, but elongated like rugby balls. These elongated receptive fields 'prefer' lines or blobs of light tilted in the same direction as their receptive field. If we represent the centre part of their receptive field as white and the surround as black, we get striped receptive fields (see figure 9.7). These receptive fields come with different tilts and sizes and positions in the overall map, each cell like the member of a vast choir, waiting to sing its note when it encounters just the right pattern in the score.

The stripy pattern of a cell's receptive field tells us the pattern of light to which it responds best. This means that we can make up a pattern or image consisting of a number of such patches, and know which set of cells will respond to it. The set of cells then becomes a 'code' for the image, and a very economical code at that, since pixel values no longer have to be specified. Patterns made up of these striped patterns look remarkably like natural textures (see figure 9.7). Mathematically, the striped patterns are called 'Gabor patches', after Nobel laureate Dennis Gabor, who described them (along with the hologram) after fleeing from Hitler to England in 1933. Each Gabor patch can be described by two numbers, one representing its tilt and the other its size. If we are using Gabor patches to describe an image, we need two further numbers to specify its map reference in the image. Four numbers, as it happens, is the same as the number of telegraphic words Galton used to describe his face profiles. In the case of textures, we can usually get away with reducing the number of words to two, by leaving out the map references. Sand remains sand even if we give it a good shaking and distribute its grains in a new random arrangement.

The receptive fields in V1 are the 'words' it uses to describe the image. Call the language 'Gaborian'. The librarians in the Babel Library of Images are delighted when they find that the books are written in Gaborian rather than in Pixelese – their catalogue becomes much simpler. Images of similar textures now stand next to one another in the catalogue. For example, the textures on the right in figure 9.7 both contain fifty patches of the same size randomly mixed with fifty patches of twice that size. The orientation and positions of the patches are random. The visual similarity between the two textures is obvious, despite their differences, and this will show up in the catalogue, because they are made from the same-sized Gabor patches. In Pixelese they would have no relationship. If we took into account the tilt of the patches, the description of the texture would be even more precise.

Another advantage of speaking Gaborian is that we immediately make an interesting discovery about natural images. The landscapes of images, it turns out, are boring and repetitive, more like East Anglia or the American Midwest than Switzerland. A mathematical law expresses the relative number of Gabor patches of each size that we expect to find, on average, in an image. Images are dominated by large patches, and this is why their landscapes are smooth, like a sandcastle that has had water poured on it. This smoothness means that 'natural images' form only a very small fraction of the number of images that are theoretically possible. We can think of images as occupying a space of many dimensions. The number of dimensions required to describe

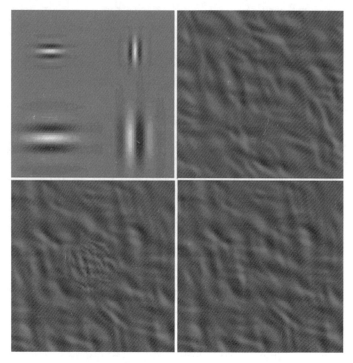

Figure 9.7 Textures made from Gabor patches

an object is the number of words required to distinguish it from other objects in the same 'space'. For example, the position of a church on an OS map can be described by two words – its grid reference. To specify that it is a church rather than a public house we need another word in the description, and thus a three-dimensional 'space'. To specify its height we need another word, and so on. The space required to describe each Babel image in Pixelese has 256 × 256 dimensions because we have to describe the intensity of every pixel separately. Neighbours in this space have similar values of pixels. In Pixelese, natural images are hopelessly scattered around this many-dimensioned space like needles in a haystack. However, in a space where each dimension is a different Gabor patch, natural images cluster together like swallowtail butterflies at the top of a hill. This is the key to understanding how the brain, or any other device, sets about making an economical catalogue for the images in the Babel Library.

Gabor receptive fields may be good at finding ridges and cliffs in image landscapes, but only in their own small patch of the image. As with motion perception, larger mechanisms are needed to see the 'big

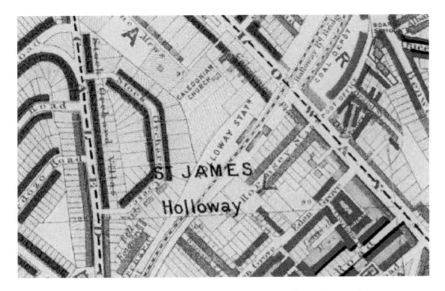

Like Minard's map, Charles Booth's 1899 'Poverty Map' of London combines topographic and non-topographic information. Different shades of colour represent the general conditions of the inhabitants of an area, with black representing the Lowest and red representing the Middle Class. This kind of representation succeeds only because people of similar condition tend to live together. Maps in the brain exploit the same tendency of similar features to cluster together in images.

The 'pinwheel map' of the visual cortex can be compared to Booth's poverty map, with colour representing the 'condition' of single cells, in this case their preference for the tilt of lines in the images on the retina. Going clockwise around each pinwheel, every tilt around the circle is represented. Preferences collapse in a 'singularity' in the centre of each pinwheel. The map is also topographic, with each pinwheel centred in a different part of the retinal image. A third form of 'condition' in the map is represented by the eye-dominance bands (black and white).

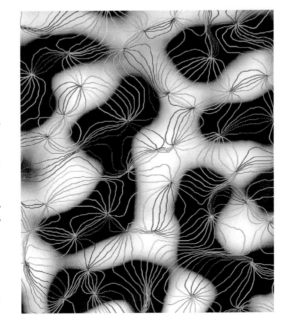

The map based on work by David van Essen and his colleagues shows how the empire of known visual areas in the macaque monkey has expanded from its original home in the primary visual cortex (V1: purple) to multiple areas in the temporal, parietal and even the frontal lobes. Quo vadis?

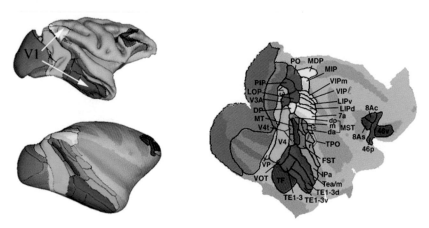

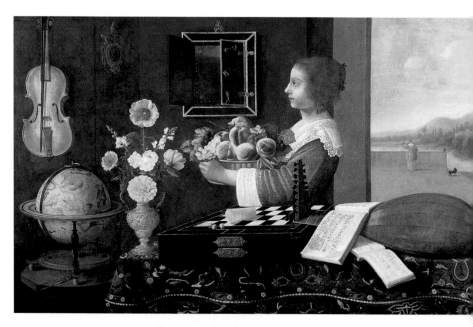

Sebastien Stoskopff's painting *Les Cinq Sens* (1633) illustrates at least six ways in which the third dimension can be represented on a flat surface.

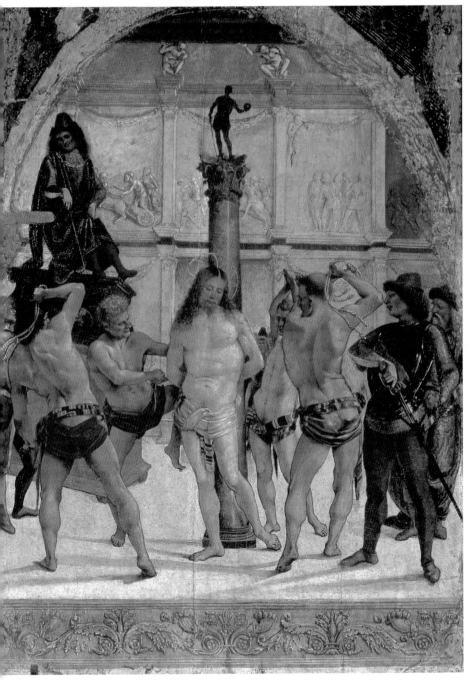

The Scourging of Christ (c. 1480) by Luca Signorelli illustrates the complexities of cast shadows on flat surfaces. The shadows from the legs of the figure on the right appear to be coming from two different light sources, but are in fact constrained to form a 'V' shape by human anatomy, here faithfully represented.

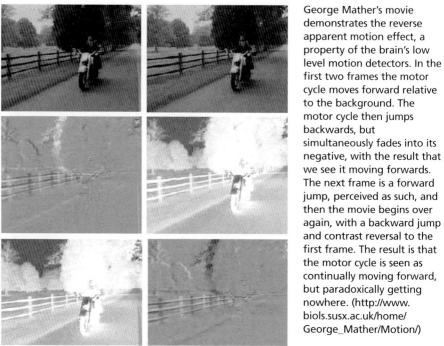

George Mather's movie demonstrates the reverse apparent motion effect, a property of the brain's low level motion detectors. In the first two frames the motor cycle moves forward relative to the background. The motor cycle then jumps backwards, but simultaneously fades into its negative, with the result that we see it moving forwards. The next frame is a forward jump, perceived as such, and then the movie begins over again, with a backward jump and contrast reversal to the first frame. The result is that the motor cycle is seen as continually moving forward, but paradoxically getting nowhere. (http://www.biols.susx.ac.uk/home/George_Mather/Motion/)

X

X

Stare fixedly at the top cross for a minute and then look at the bottom cross. The yellow discs to the left and right of the cross will appear tinged with green and red respectively: the complimentary colours to the red and green discs to which the eye has become adapted.

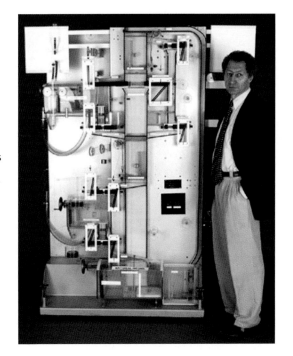

The analogue computer built by Bill Phillips of the London School of Economics represented the flow of money around the economy by the movement of coloured liquid around Perspex pipes.

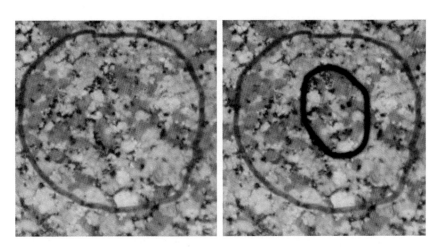

The opium-eating de Quincy was afflicted by what he called 'the tyranny of the human face'. Even without opium, we have such a powerful schema of the face that we see it in random images, like the 'Man in the Moon' or (as here) in a granite pavement.

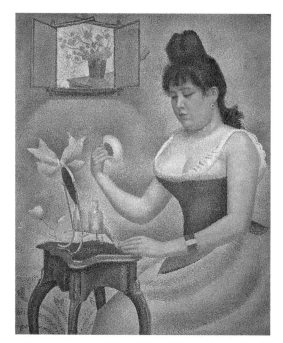

George Seurat's *La Poudreuse* (1890) is composed, like computer images, of many small picture elements or 'pixels'. Seurat (a keen follower of visual science) discovered that the meaning of images can be discerned even when the pixels are large enough to be visually resolved as separate elements.

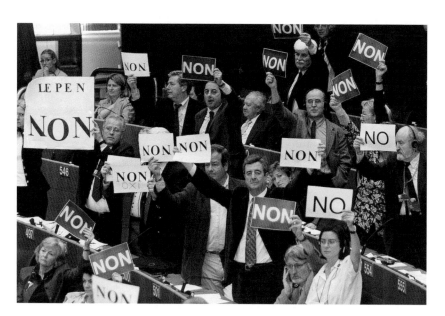

At a protest in the European Parliament, several deputies are betrayed by their serifs. Their signs are upside down. But how does our brain know which way is 'up' – by the inverted image on the retina, or by gravity?

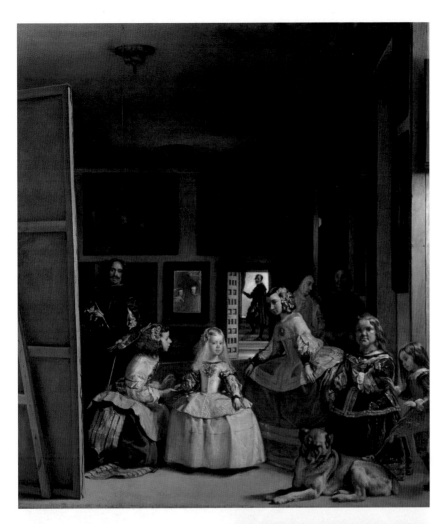

Las Meninas by Velázquez (1656) refutes the common misconception that mirrors reverse left and right. The mirror at the back of the room reflects the images of the couple (otherwise invisible) that are the subject of the painter's attention. To appear on the right-hand side of the mirror, Philip IV would have to be standing facing the mirror to the right of his wife. There is no optical reversal.

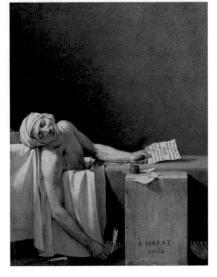

David's depiction of the assassination of Jean-Paul Marat, the only writer of a book on consciousness (*Philosophical Essay on Man*, 1773) to have got his just deserts.

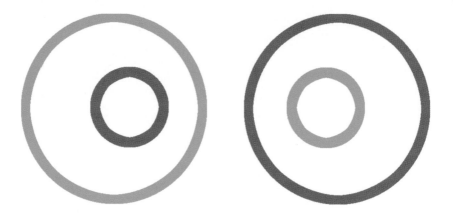

This image by Anne Treisman shows that stable binocular depth perception can exist at the same time as alternating colour rivalry. Most beginners find these figures very difficult to fuse. One method is to hold the page very close to the eye and to use a playing card held vertically so that the left eye figure is visible only to the left eye, and the right eye figure by the right eye. After a few seconds the two images should fuse into one. The image will be blurred, but if the page is then gradually distanced from the eye, it should get sharper while remaining single.

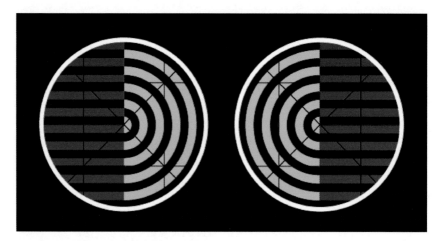

The figure, originating with Diaz-Caneja, is held to show that the images from the two eyes are combined to produce shape *before* rather than after 'binocular rivalry'. When the two images are fused by squinting, observers tend to see completed green/black rings alternating with completed red/black stripes. However, a large variety of other perceptions are reported, in which one or other eye dominates.

picture'. To respond selectively to a texture, a single cell would need a large receptive field, getting its input from cells with smaller receptive fields. The cells form a hierarchy, small reporting to large, like the angelic hierarchy of the Areopagite, which contained three divisions of angels, each one with three orders (the cherubim, for example). In a hierarchy, each member reports to the next level up, and this is the idea behind a hierarchy of feature detectors. A receptive field in V1 is already a high-ranking member of a hierarchy, because it receives and filters reports from many thousands of cones in the retina, through the divisions of optic nerve fibres and cells in the thalamus; but the process could continue. Several cells in V1 could report to a single cell in V2, and so on to higher levels: 'Big fleas have little fleas / Upon their backs to bite 'em. / The little fleas have smaller fleas / And so on *infinitum.*'

The highest-ranking members of the hierarchy discovered so far are in the temporal lobe of the monkey. Cells in the lower part of the temporal lobe have 'preferences' for real objects, such as hands and faces, or even for particular faces, even if the face is presented from different viewpoints. These cells are not particularly interested in the exact size or position of their preferred object on the retina: they seem to have solved one of the Babel librarians' biggest problems. Of course, we cannot conclude from this that single cells cause our awareness of a face or hand; it is likely that a cell responding to a face will in fact be responding to a collection of simple 'features' such as two circles and a horizontal line, representing eyes and mouth. Other cells would almost certainly be involved in awareness of the face, including those responding to texture and 3-D geometry. Detailed study of cells with object preferences often show that they respond to simple geometric shapes or their combination. Remarkably, one experiment says that cells with similar shape preferences cluster together in vertical columns, like those in the primary visual cortex.

The hierarchical theory says that cells in the temporal lobe get their elaborate shape preferences by combining simpler features from cells lower down in the hierarchy. Eventually, the theory goes, the messages go up the hierarchy until we get cells that report a particular individual's face: 'face recognition cells', or 'grandmother cells', as they are called in the trade. The theory is appealing to those who like hierarchies, but it has logical problems. Suppose we did find a single cell that responds to Grandmother's face, and to no other. The buck could not stop there. How could the firing of a single cell just by itself give rise to the complex experience of a person? Such a cell would have to have an output to other parts of the brain that could retrieve the name of the face, its emotional expression, its friends and so on. So the hierarch needs now to report to a whole set of lower orders. Why, then, bother to have a hierarch at all? Why not go directly from a set of lower level 'features', like those actually found in the 'columns' of the temporal lobe, to the large set of nerve cells representing the concept of the person? This would be a neural network rather than a hierarchy. In the neural network theory, face recognition is not found in a single archangel, but is distributed around a network of many cherubim. Neural networks are appealing to people who dislike hierarchies. As far as the temporal lobe is concerned, hierarchs and networkers are still slugging it out.

The late Maurice Bowra liked to confuse people by saying, 'I know your name, but I can't remember your face.' (This is the same fellow of All Souls who defined the collective name for the heads of Oxford colleges as 'a lack of principles'.) Bowra apart, we often forget names, but seldom forget a face. Why? One theory is that face recognition cells can fire even when their links to names have been forgotten. If these face recognition cells are clustered together in one part of the brain, they might be vulnerable to brain damage; and indeed, some brain-damaged patients have great difficulty in recognising faces. They cannot even name famous people such as Winston Churchill from their faces, although they can tell you what the person is famous for, if told their name. This condition (called 'prosopagnosia') is caused by damage to visual areas outside the primary visual cortex, located near the boundary between the occipital and temporal lobes. Functional brain imaging has identified two main regions (the 'fusiform face area' and the inferior occipital gyrus) where there is particularly strong activity when the observer is looking at faces. Prosopagnosia is usually associated with brain injury, but some people lack the ability to recognise faces from birth. The 'face areas' in the brains of these 'developmental prosopagnosics', as they are called, are no more responsive to faces than to other objects, such as hands.

Prosopagnosia was originally thought to affect only recognition of human faces. A different interpretation is that the patient has lost the ability to make very fine discriminations. One single-case study tells of a farmer who lost the ability to distinguish between his sheep after brain damage; another is the case of an ornithologist who lost the ability to distinguish between similar birds, like the blackbird and the ring ouzel. So there may not be a specialised 'face area' in the brain at all, but rather an area where practice has made perfect. The latest evidence from functional brain imaging shows that the so-called face area is the tip of a much larger iceberg, where there is particularly intense activity during face recognition. Recognition of faces, houses and chairs causes peaks of activity in slightly different regions of the fusiform face area, but all of them cause widespread and overlapping activity over nearby regions. Just looking at peaks in maps can be misleading. Charles Booth's map of poverty street by street in London shows a peak in the East End, but there was plenty of poverty elsewhere.

The 'face area' also responds to cartoons of faces, and to caricatures. Caricatures are to vision what parody is to literature. The point of literary parody is to copy the style of the original but to exaggerate its ludicrous aspects. One of the most parodied poems in the English language is 'Excelsior', by Longfellow, in which the young hero climbs the highest mountain to his inevitable death, clutching a banner with the word 'Excelsior!' A parody by Edward Lear substitutes a porker, who duly meets a dreadful fate:

> There in the twilight, cold and grey
> Lifeless but beautiful he lay
> And solemn voices seemed to say
> Fresh pork and sausages today
> Excelsior!

It is a nice question whether parodies and their originals in the Babel Library could be classified together on the basis of similarity. A really clever parody should be as unlike the original as possible on the surface, while immediately suggesting its origin. (In this sense, Lear's parody is not that good). A parody can be of a style rather than of a particular book, like Flann O'Brien's send-up of the heroic Celtic in 'At Swim Two Birds'. A simple matching of words will not necessarily detect a good parody. The same problem will arise in the Image Library with caricature. Caricatures are interesting because they are images that are very different from their originals in Pixelese, but just as easy to recognise, and sometimes even more so. How can this be, if there are special 'face cells' sitting around in the brain waiting for their own favourite face to come along? They should respond best to the normal face they have seen before, not to a caricature. The heir to the English throne does not really have ears as large as those of an African elephant. Caricatures exaggerate the original. If Michelle Pfeiffer has her eyes farther apart than most people, you can be sure that a caricature will put them further apart still. None of this squares with the idea that the brain recognises faces by matching them with some simple memory of previous images. Something more elaborate must be involved.

Francis Galton, once again, gave us the right way to think about the problem of caricature. He added together the images of a large number of faces to produce the 'average face'. Average faces look quite beautiful in an insipid sort of way, because the averaging irons out the normal asymmetries of the human face and removes blemishes such as small-pox scars. Darwinian psychologists say that symmetrical faces are sexually attractive because they indicate superior genes. (Have these psychologists never heard of beauty spots or experienced the fatal attraction of heterochromia – differently coloured left and right eyes?) Caricatures exaggerate differences from the average face. The first step in caricaturing a face is to observe what distinguishes it from the average face. Perhaps it has a slightly longer nose and slightly bushier eyebrows. Make the nose longer still and the eyebrows even bushier and you have a caricature. A skilled caricaturist is adept at detecting small differences from the average and accentuating them. It is as if we have a concept of the average face somewhere in our brain.

Galton also produced average faces of groups such as clergymen and criminals of various sorts. He evidently hoped by this to refute King Duncan's claim that 'There's no art / To find the mind's construction in the face.' Galton hoped that average images would help in rounding up the usual suspects. Perhaps, in the end, average burglars could have their offending genes removed from the gene pool. Alas for eugenics, the idea did not work, for the face of the average burglar is no different from the average clergyman. Duncan was right after all. It is unhelpful to describe a face as one-quarter burglar and three-quarters clergyman; much more helpful, as it turns out, is to describe each face as a mixture of the average face, and a small number of other face-like images that make the face different from the average. For historical reasons best known to mathematicians, these building blocks for faces are called 'eigenfaces' (see figure 9.8). It turns out that as few as a dozen of these face-like images are enough to make passable likenesses of several thousand faces. In other words, faces can be described in a much, much smaller space than the space needed to describe all images – not surprising, since faces are all very much alike.

Eigenfaces can be used to make caricatures. In 'face space', a particular face is represented as a point, and there will be a line or vector

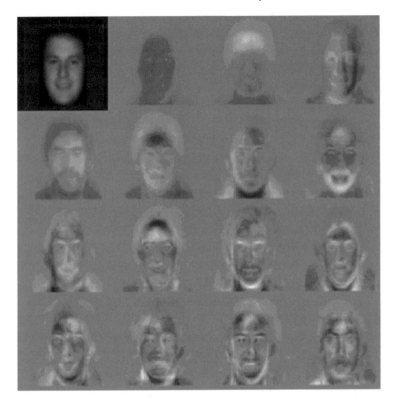

Figure 9.8 Eigenfaces

that joins it to the average face in the middle of the space. Other faces will lie nearby at greater or lesser distances. Faces near to the average face will all lie very close together and will be difficult to distinguish, especially in the presence of ubiquitous 'noise'. However, faces far away from the average will have fewer neighbours and will be easier to distinguish. Caricature pushes a face further away from the average, and thus makes it more distinctive. It will be easier to recognise which vector it lies on, and thus its identity, if it is pushed further out in the space, away from similar faces.

For every caricature there is an anti-caricature on the opposite side of face space, like the two planets in Isaac Asimov's 'Foundation Trilogy', which had mirror-image positions and cultures. The caricature and its anti-caricature are joined by a straight line (in face space) that passes through the average face. If the caricature has an eagle beak like the Duke of Wellington, the anti-caricature has a snub nose. The anti-caricature of Michelle Pfeiffer has her eyes close together, like Tony

Blair's. Presumably, if we lived in a world where most people had their eyes very wide apart, we should see them as normal, and Tony Blair as a caricature. An experiment with computer-generated caricatures has put this idea to the test. Observers learned to discriminate 'Adam' from 'Jim' or 'Henry' (see figure 9.9). Shown the average face and asked whether it was Adam or Jim, they were, unsurprisingly, unable to make a consistent choice. However, if they were first 'adapted' to 'Anti-Adam' by staring at his image for several minutes, and then shown the average face, they were confident that it was Adam. The experiment recalls the 'waterfall effect', in which staring at downwards-flowing motion causes stationary stimuli to appear flowing upwards. Like the waterfall effect, the face experiment suggests that we base our decisions on the balance between opposites.

We have come a long way from Pixelese. The brain represents shapes and textures in an abstract space of many dimensions, where the dimensions are 'features'. The retina begins the process of translating Pixelese into Gaborian – the language of the primary visual cortex.

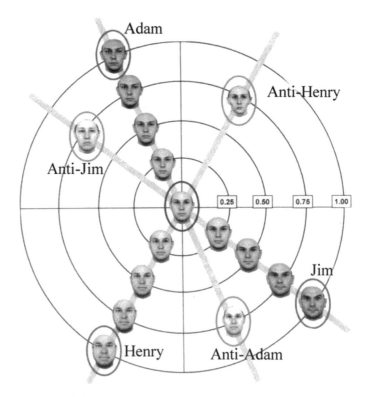

Figure 9.9 Faces and their 'Anti-Faces'

This is followed by specialised representations, such as face space. However, these spaces of many dimensions are very different from the topographical maps like the map in the primary visual cortex, and they have their limitations. Face space might tell us that a particular face has an unusually large nose, but it would be no help in reaching out to touch that nose. To find the regions of the brain where perception is linked to space and action we need to arrest our descent into the temporal lobe and move upwards instead into the parietal lobe.

PART THREE
SPACE AND THE BODY

10

'Whirling madly through the darkness'

We can close our eyes and imagine the space around us, and rearrange imagined objects around our body. One of the best descriptions of these mental gymnastics is in the opening chapter of Marcel Proust's *Swann's Way*, where the narrator is waking up in bed without knowing at first where he is:

> For it always happened that when I awoke like this, and my mind struggled in an unsuccessful attempt to discover where I was, everything would be moving about me through the darkness: things, places, years. My body, still too heavy with sleep to move, would make an effort to construe the form which its tiredness took as an orientation of its various members, so as to induce from that where the wall lay and the furniture stood, to piece together and give a name to the house in which it must be living. Its memory, the composite memory of its ribs, knees and shoulder blades offered it a whole series of rooms in which it had at one time or another slept; while the unseen walls kept changing, adapting themselves to the shape of each successive room that it remembered, whirling madly through the darkness. (Proust, *Swann's Way*)

Objects are moved about in imagination until they occupy the correct relation to the body. Sometimes one has the annoying feeling that objects are in the wrong place in the invisible room: the window that should be behind the head is in front. The room seems to spin in the darkness, and order is restored.

The space in which the walls and furniture are 'whirling madly' is defined by our body. Although our body stops at the skin, it imposes itself on the objects around it. The space we inhabit is not the same in all directions, like the space of physics, but quite different in character in different directions – for example, in front of us and behind. Space behind us is perceived, and can be occupied by someone in a seat behind us, making us uncomfortable by staring at our neck, but it is shadowy and compressed in comparison to the space in front. Even the shape of objects is not defined without reference to the body. An upside-down image of a famous face is much harder to recognise than one the right way up. Expressions are particularly hard to read, as Wittgenstein pointed out: 'Hold a drawing of a face upside down and you can't recognise the expression of the face. Perhaps you can see that it is smiling, but not exactly what kind of smile it is. You cannot imitate the smile or describe it more exactly' (*Philosophical Investigations*, II, xi).

Because we use the same word, 'space', to describe an aspect of our perception and the world described by physics, it is easy to confuse the two. However, the space that we experience through our bodies could not be more different from the silent and empty spaces between the stars. We should look to Proust rather than to Newton or Einstein for our experience of space. Statements like the following make sense to a physicist :

- The magnetic permeability of empty space is $4\pi \times 10^{-7}$ henrys per metre
- The permittivity of empty space is 8.55×10^{-12} farads per metre

The book from which these two examples are taken goes on to give twenty-two properties of physical space in all, including the fact that space is curved. For many of us these statements are difficult to understand. How can the absence of anything have properties? How can nothing have a number like 8.55×10^{-12} farads attached to it? We perceive space as a relation between objects, not as something that has properties in its own right. If we experience a space between objects A and B we mean that a line drawn between them would have a certain length, or that, to move our eyes from one to the other, we should have to move them in a certain direction (relative to our body) and for a certain distance. That purely empty space could have physical properties, or that it could be curved, defeats our perceptual imagination. When light was found to travel through 'empty' space as waves, a superfluous ether was invented as a sop to intuition.

The ether was finally abolished by Michelson and Morley's famous experiment in Chicago. But the powerful lure of spatial intuition makes us try to translate the physical properties of space into statements about relations between objects. The best that can be said about these efforts is that they are cumbersome. The permittivity of 8.55×10^{-12} farads per metre of empty space has to be replaced by a lengthy statement about interactions between objects and measuring instruments. In a similar vein, the French physicist Henri Poincaré objected to the statement that space was curved. Poincaré said that if experiment found that the sum of the interior angles of a triangle formed by light rays was greater than 180 degrees, it would be simpler to say that light does not travel in straight lines than to say that space is curved. Logically, this 'conventionalist' position, as it is called, cannot be refuted, but nor can the proposition that the Earth is flat, if one is prepared to be sufficiently subtle about it. Physicists have, by and large, ignored Poincaré's conventionalism, finding it simpler to assume that space itself has physical properties, unlike the space of our perception. In April 2002, the first-round result of the French Presidential Election led the newspaper *Figaro* to take up most of its front page with the single word 'Séisme' (Earthquake). The far-right candidate Jean-Marie Le Pen obtained 18 per cent of the popular vote to beat the Prime Minister, of the Socialist Party, into third place. Demonstrations against Le Pen followed in several large French towns, members of the European Parliament in Brussels jeered Le Pen as he entered the chamber and held up signs saying 'NON'. The only problem was that some of the signs were held upside down (see plate section). The inversion can be recognised in the asymmetrical typefaces with serifs. One demonstrator has managed to get his left 'N' the wrong way up and the other the right way round. Luckily, the English 'NOs' in the photograph are held the right way up. 'NON' are unusual in being both a palindrome and composed of letters that look the same upside down. If instead we take the headline above the photograph and invert it, we see:

Bɹnssǝʅs sɐʎs ᴎou ʇo ꞁǝ Ԁǝu

The message is difficult to read. But is that because it is upside down on the eye, upside down with respect to the head, or because it is inverted with respect to gravity? Why should its orientation matter at all? Computers would not care if text were inverted: they could invert it in a microsecond. The brain is clearly different. Orientation with respect to the body matters, and orientation gives its peculiar flavour to our subjective space.

In physical space, an object remains the same object when it is rotated. Not so for us. If we see two objects side by side and have to decide whether they are the same or different, it is harder if one of the objects is rotated relative to the other. Which cartoon face in figure 10.1 has the same eye open as the centre version? It takes a few moments to tell. Experiments like these on 'mental rotation' have shown that the time it takes to compare two rotated objects increases with the angle of rotation between them. There would be no reason for this if the objects were described in a frame of reference independent of our body. Suppose that, as in the figure, the part of the face containing the mouth were labelled 'S', and 'N', 'E' and 'W' filled in accordingly. The problem of deciding whether the black eye is on the same side of the head then becomes a simple one of deciding whether they are both 'W'. They are, so the faces are the same. Clearly, our brain does not perform the task in this way. We describe the black eye in the upright face as on the right (relative to our body) and we then have to decide whether it would be on our left or on our right in the other face if it were rotated to the upright. The imagining of the rotation takes time, as if we have to reconstruct a description of the face at intermediate angles. This does not mean that an image is being rotated in our head: imagining a rotation is not the same as rotating an image. Imagining a rotation means constructing a new description of the image, in the axes of our own body.

Map reading depends on mental rotation, and this may be why some people find it difficult. If one is driving south, towns to the left of the road on the map are on the right-hand side of the car, but an experienced navigator does not have to turn the road atlas upside down to know which way to turn at a road junction. However, many people prefer to

Figure 10.1 Mental rotation

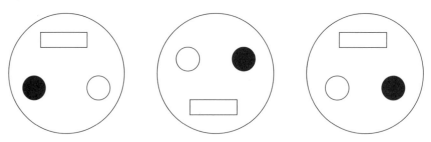

have a map oriented so that a left turn will be on their left-hand side, and they will turn a map upside down to make it so. It is even possible to buy upside-down maps of London with North at the bottom of the page, presumably for the use of people who have the misfortune of being obliged to visit South London from the North. People prefer a particular relation between a map and their own body: they like a left turn to be represented on the left side of the map.

Sometimes a reference frame changes spontaneously, and we perceive a figure changing its orientation without any physical change in the image. The simplest of all reversible figures is an image of several equilateral triangles, all pointing in the same direction. There are three possible perceptual interpretations, depending on which vertex of the triangle we choose to be the pointing direction. The change that happens when the triangles 'flip' direction is very hard to describe, but just as unmistakable as the 'flip' of the Necker cube. In physical space, of course, the triangles have no direction: the change that we perceive when they flip is a change in their description relative to our body. It is interesting that all the triangles flip together, suggesting that the description of their direction applies to all of them. We get the same 'flip' when looking at a rotating weathervane or anemometer with one eye closed; the direction of rotation spontaneously reverses from clockwise to anticlockwise. Laboratory experiments have shown that if there are several of these ambiguous objects in the field of view, they all change direction simultaneously.

Our skill at mental rotation is responsible for the widespread but mistaken belief that mirrors reverse left and right. A mirror in my study shows the reflection of a poster on the opposite wall with the text:

ʞoʞoɘɔɥɒʞ *bⁿɒ Scotland*

and underneath these words is the recognisable 'Still Life with marrow, bean and golden yellow leaf (1945)', the right side up. The mirror appears to have inverted left and right without inverting up and down. But if instead of looking at a painting in a mirror we look at the representation of a mirror in a painting – for example in Velasquez' *Las Meninas* (see plate section) – we immediately see that a mirror inverts neither up/down nor left/right. King Philip IV and his wife Mariana are invisible except in the mirror, but we know from the laws of optics that the King is on the right-hand side of the canvas from our point of view, as is his image in the mirror. As an outsider to the scene we can see that the mirror has reversed nothing. For the painter, the King is on the left-hand side of the canvas, as is the reflection of the King in the mirror. There is no reversal here.

The apparent problem of reversal arises only when we use the mirror to read something behind us, or when we hold up a page of print between us and the mirror. In the latter case we turn the paper through 180 degrees around a vertical axis to present it to the mirror. It is this rotation that reverses left and right relative to our body, not the mirror. If instead we present the page to the mirror by rotating it 180 degrees around a horizontal axis, we reverse up and down but not left and right. As for the poster on the wall behind us, we have reversed left and right relative to our body by turning our back on it in order to look at the mirror. If instead we look at the mirror through our legs, as an old custom enjoins the Japanese to do when looking at a mountain, something very curious indeed happens. The text is no longer left–right reversed but is oddly difficult to read. Close inspection reveals that it is upside down (look at the position of the descenders and ascenders).

The mystery of the mirror is not that it reverses left and right but that anyone should ever have thought that it did. There must be a psychological explanation for our puzzlement about mirrors, and the obvious one is unconscious mental rotation. When we look at ourselves in the mirror we see our reflection looking back at us, which it is easy to perceive as another person behind the mirror. If we raise our right hand, the 'person' behind the mirror raises a hand on the right-hand side of our body; but by mental rotation we can see that this would be the left hand of the person in the mirror. Thus we say that the mirror has reversed left and right, but we are mistaken: the reversal has been done by our act of mental rotation.

We seem to have solved the problem of mirror reversal, but not quite. If we look at text reflected in a mirror, but through our legs, the text is inverted and difficult to read; but does the whole scene seem inverted? Do the Japanese see Fuji-San upside down through their legs? Different observers might have different impressions here, but the impression of the writer is that objects such as chairs do not seem upside down. Moreover, if one points first to the real top of the object and then to the bottom, the feeling is that the arm has moved downwards in space, as indeed it has with respect to gravity. (We can define an experimental psychologist, at this point, as someone who looks at the world through a mirror with his head upside down and wonders why the world is not seen upside down.) The brain has information about gravity from gravity-sensitive organs in the ear called the otoliths. This may explain why the world does not look upside down when we look at it through our legs. Trees still point upwards in the gravitational frame, even if their images have been upended on the retina. But if this is so, why is the text so difficult to read? We begin to suspect at this point that there is not a single reference frame for vision. The recognition of text and faces takes place in a retinal frame, but for deciding whether objects are upright or not, we rely to some extent at least on gravity. Trees do not seem to tilt off the vertical when we tilt our head.

Swift's 'Big-Endians' and 'Little-Endians' in *Gulliver's Travels* fought over the correct way of opening an egg. This was irrational, but is it any more obvious why faces and text have to be 'the right way up' before we recognise them? Perhaps the brain mechanisms responsible for their recognition are highly specialised for speed and do not have time to consider all possible orientations. In other words, they are specialised analogue computers, with an orientation of their own. Experiments on reading show that there is indeed a speed-reading mechanism, sensitive to orientation. Reading is not one skill, but at least two. The most obvious way to read is to recognise the letters individually and spell them out to form the word, like 'C - A - M'. Even this simple letter-by-letter strategy depends on a frame of reference. 'CAM' is not the same as 'CAW', but 'M' is very similar to a rotated 'W'. We also have to read the text in the correct direction: left to right in English, right to left in Hebrew, and up down in some forms of Chinese. In the Ancient Greek text known as boustrophedon ('as an ox turns in ploughing'), alternate lines were read from left to right and right to left; the reader of boustrophedon presumably had a moment of hesitation reading a single line drawn randomly from a script, while deciding whether to scan left to right or right to left. If text is inverted, by turning the page upside down or by looking at it in a mirror, we have to scan it in the unaccustomed direction, and evidently the brain finds this difficult. Mirror-writing is a particularly interesting case, because the direction of scanning is reversed, without turning the text upside down. It is possible with practice to produce mirror writing, particularly with the left hand if one is right-handed, and to read it quite quickly. The best-known mirror writer is Leonardo da Vinci, whose reasons for writing backwards have been much debated.

We normally distinguish between 'perception' as an input to our brain, and 'action' as an output; but reading shows how artificial the distinction can be. Reading is a skill like playing the piano, except that we move our eyes instead of our hands and fingers. (An inexperienced reader will even enlist a moving finger.) The action of reading requires a frame of reference, and this frame seems to be the eye itself, rather than an external frame such as gravity.

Most of us, though perhaps not some kinds of dyslexics, progress beyond letter-by-letter reading to the faster skill of reading by 'word shape' :

iFyOuNeEdEvIdEnCeTrYReAdInGtHiS

When word shape is abolished by alternating upper/lower case and leaving out the spaces, reading is laborious. On the other hand, we can blur text to the point where individual letter recognition becomes difficult, and still have a good shot at recognising the words, as in figure 10.2.

The shape of a word is defined by its length, by its pattern of descenders and ascenders, and by variations in density. Perhaps ascenders and descenders were invented to give words more recognisable shapes; certainly, text composed entirely in upper case is more difficult to read. The earliest texts in Greek and Latin did not have spaces between the words, leading to the interesting idea that readers of these texts had not yet invented the word-shape method of reading. If this is so, they were in the position of some stroke victims, who appear to have lost word-shape reading, although they can still read letter by letter. They will read 'Pint' as if it rhymes with 'Lint'. Other patients will read 'Pint' correctly but not made-up words like 'Gint': they have lost letter-by-letter reading.

In Italian, irregularities such as 'pint' and 'lint' are almost unknown. Bernard Shaw wanted to reform English spelling to make it easier, and would have been delighted by research showing that Italians suffer less than Anglo-Saxons from the effects of dyslexia. Dyslexia is still a

Figure 10.2 Blurred text and letters. The words on top are legible; the letters below are not.

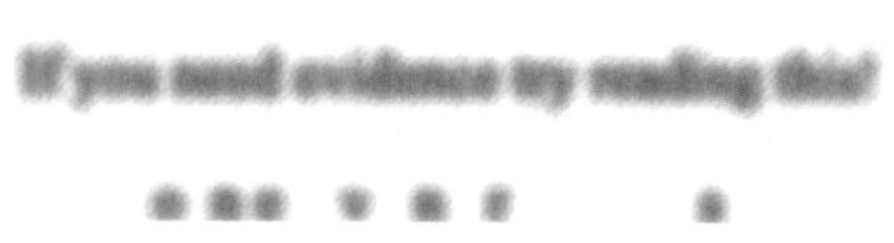

controversial subject, but it is not confined to the children of middle-class parents, as saloon-bar pundits like to proclaim. It is recognised scientifically as a condition in which the child's performance on the verbal sections of IQ tests are much lower than those on the spatial components. A biological basis for the condition is supported by the fact that it is considerably more common in males than females, but just as common in Italian children as in Anglo-Saxons, provided the same sensitive measures are used.

Dyslexia is not a single condition. Some dyslexics are persuaded that their reading is improved by wearing rose-tinted spectacles, but it is not easy to distinguish this from a placebo effect. On the other hand, a problem in building up sounds from letters ('grapheme to phoneme conversion') is suggested by the difficulty many dyslexic children have with Spoonerisms. Given the classic Spoonerism: 'You have hissed all my mystery lectures and must leave Oxford by the town drain,' or the phrase 'Erotic Blacks' in a geology lecture, many dyslexics find the decoding difficult. Dr Spooner himself suffered from a peculiar neurological condition for which there is no recognised name; according to one anecdote he spilt some salt on the table and immediately poured his glass of claret over it to save the tablecloth. His speech problem seems to have been part of a more general difficulty in getting actions in their correct order. The American physician Samuel Orton thought that the core problem for dyslexics was that they were unsure about left and right. Orton coined the ugly term 'strephosymbolia' (twisted letters) to describe the alleged tendency of dyslexics to confuse their 'b's and 'd's and to read words backwards or in a jumbled order. The apocryphal story of the dyslexic who sold his soul to Santa supports Orton's conjecture, but there is little scientific evidence that 'strephosymbolia' is the main problem in dyslexia.

A different kind of dyslexia is sometimes seen in the neurological syndrome of 'parietal neglect', which may have afflicted the novelist Charles Dickens. Dickens was apparently a keen reader of *The Lancet* and would have been interested in an article 'Charles Dickens: a neglected diagnosis', published in the December issue of the journal in 2001. The article relates that Dickens described to his future biographer John Forster a peculiar state of vision he had observed in the signs over shops: 'He told us that as he came along, walking up the length of Oxford Street, the same incident had recurred as on the day of a former dinner with us, and that he had not been able to read, all the way, more than the right-hand half of the names over the shops.'

Dickens also suffered from odd feelings in his left leg and of 'strangeness' in his left hand. His symptoms became worse after his experience of the catastrophic train derailment at Staplehurst on 9 June 1865. The permanent-way gang replacing timber baulks on the Beult viaduct miscalculated the arrival time of the 'tidal' boat train from Folkestone, the only train not to have a fixed place in the timetable, for obvious reasons. Two 21-foot lengths of rail were still missing when the express arrived, shot over the gap, and derailed the following coaches, in one of which Dickens was reading the manuscript of *Our Mutual Friend*. He was unable to travel by train comfortably after that, and had a strange 'conviction against the senses' that trains were leaning to the left side. As with his hand and leg, it was the left side of the train that was affected, and all this is consistent with problems in the right side of the brain. In his classic book *Red for Danger*, L. T. C. Rolt says, 'We cannot estimate the loss which English Literature sustained as a result of John Benge's tragic mistake. Certainly he deprived us of the solution to *The Mystery of Edwin Drood*.' This may be to overestimate both the influence of the crash and the solubility of the uncompleted plot, but certainly Dickens died from a stroke very soon afterwards; no post mortem was carried out, so we do not know which area of the brain was affected by the earlier premonitions.

Dickens may have been suffering from the neurological condition called 'neglect dyslexia' associated with damage to the lower part of the parietal lobe, particularly on the right-hand side of the brain. Patients with 'spatial neglect' tend to ignore one half of visual space, most usually the left-hand side if they are right-handed (as Dickens was). They may ignore a person who enters from the left side of their space, and to all intents and purposes behave as if the left side of space were non-existent. 'Neglect dyslexia' is a specific form applying to reading. Dickens did not say whether he was unable to read the left-hand side of shop signs, or one side of his retina. However, we can guess from other patients that his blind area did not move when he moved his eyes (unlike Wollaston, who was blind to the right of *'the spot to which my eyes were directed'*). In a standard diagnostic test of neglect, the patient is asked to cross out every line or letter 'A' that he can find on a sheet of paper (see figure 10.3). He succeeds in crossing out all the 'A's on the right-hand side of the page but apparently fails to notice those on the left. This is most unlikely to be the result of not seeing the image on one side of the retina, since the patient is free to move his eyes all around the page. If the eyes were moved to the left-hand side of the sheet, all the letters would now fall in the right-hand side of the visual field, and should become visible. This could be explained by a retinal blindness if the patient never in fact moves his eyes to the left of the body midline; but even this hypothesis would not explain why a neglect patient asked to draw a flower from memory puts leaves and petals on the right-hand side only. Clearly, neglect does not depend only on the position of the image in the eye. Apparently, the direction in which the limbs and trunk of the body are pointing are more important than the direction of gaze. This is confirmed by asking the patient to move his head and body while continuing to gaze in the same direction. Objects that have previously been neglected because they were located on the left-hand side of the body are now noticed.

Patients with neglect sometimes ignore parts of the body when they are dressing, or even apply make-up to the right side of the face alone. 'Dressing neglect' can hardly be due to an area of blindness on one side of the eye, since we typically look at our shoes when trying to put them on. Neglect can even apply in the imagination. An Italian patient,

Figure 10.3 Parietal neglect syndrome

A
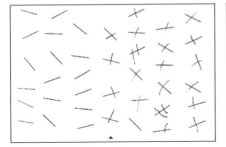
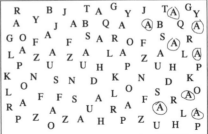

B

C
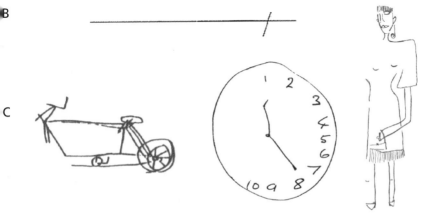

asked to imagine the Piazza de Duomo in Milan from two opposite viewpoints, described the buildings on the right-hand side of the imaged scene, but omitted those on the left. When asked to describe the scene from the other side of the Piazza the patient again described only the buildings on the right; but these were, of course, a different set from those described in the earlier scene. The patient's memory for the buildings was clearly intact, but could be retrieved only from the correct vantage point, rather as we fail to identify our dentist when we meet him in the supermarket. Another patient taken to the Piazza de Duomo had difficulties in navigating towards locations on his left-hand side:

> With his back to the Cathedral, he had no trouble in making for locations to his right, such as La Scala. However, he appeared completely disoriented when asked to head for locations to his left; for instance, he could not bend towards Via Torino (to the left), kept saying that he knew it was near there and was baffled by his failures. Moreover, his first hesitant steps to a given location he was asked to head for were towards the right.

Not all neglect patients show all of these symptoms; the syndrome is highly complicated, and no two patients are identical. Some patients show no neglect of objects on the left-hand side until competing objects are present on the right. Asked how many fingers they see when the investigator holds up both index fingers they say 'one'; but they make the same response when only the left-hand finger is held up. Clearly, they are not 'blind' at all in the ordinary sense of the word; but when objects are simultaneously present on both left and right they act as if only the one on the right is present. We can get some insight into how this feels by getting two people to read to us out loud, one into our left ear and the other into the right. By carefully attending to one side of space (left or right) we can hear what is being said to the complete exclusion of the message to the other ear. Experiences of this kind show that very little of the message in the 'unattended' ear gets through to consciousness. Similarities like these have led to the suggestion that neglect is caused by an extreme failure of attention to the left-hand side of space.

The explanation is unhelpful without a definition of attention. William James (1842–1910), in probably the best book ever written on the topic (*The Principles of Psychology*, 1890), said that attention was 'the taking possession by the mind, in a clear and vivid form, of one of what may seem simultaneously possible objects or trains of thought'. In other words, attention resolves potential conflicts, either in perception, thought or action. Pathological lack of attention has been implicated in all sorts of neurological and psychiatric conditions – even in the failure of 'neurasthenic' young men (ruined by vicious practices in school) to listen to lectures: 'The most general complaint of these men is of incapability to follow the thought of the Professor for something less than an hour without having their attention distracted, or to maintain a determined order of ideas in consciousness for a desirable length of time' (Bianchi's *Textbook of Psychiatry*, 1906).

Indeed. But what is this 'attention'? Perhaps it would be better to turn the question round, and ask whether the symptoms of neglect throw any new light on the brain mechanisms of attention. A starting point is the observation that neglect of a particular region can be overcome by turning the body towards the previously neglected side of space. Also, many neglect patients are slow and reluctant to reach for objects in the neglected region, even using their preferred hand (the right). Even more interestingly, some neglect patients can have specific neglect for objects within reaching range, while others neglect only objects that are out of reach. Reaching includes tool use, so that a patient with 'near' neglect might neglect the left-hand side of a dartboard when throwing darts, or reaching for objects with a stick. These facts tell us that there is a strong link between neglect, attention and action.

The idea that there is an intimate relation between perceived space and action is not new: philosophers such as Berkeley speculated that our concept of space is closely related to our ability to move and to manipulate objects. A possible solution to the puzzle of neglect is that parts of the parietal lobe are closely involved in the use of vision to guide action. When these are damaged, areas of personal space 'disappear' because the ability to direct action into these areas has become impaired. One idea is that regions of the parietal lobe are involved in transforming between different 'frames of reference' when we move parts or all of our bodies. These transformations are the topic of the next chapter.

11

Frames of Reference

By the 1870s the long task of finding out which parts of the brain do what was well under way. In 1861 Paul Broca, in France, had discovered a language centre in the left frontal lobe of one of his patients – 'Tan', so called because this was the only word he could utter after his brain injury. In 1870, the year of the Franco-Prussian war and the Paris Commune, Fritsch and Hitzig showed that a weak electric current applied to a small part of the frontal cortex of a dog produced movement of the limbs on the opposite side of the body. They had discovered the motor cortex, damage to which in man produces paralysis of voluntary movement. The search was now on for the parts of the brain responsible for perception, especially for the visual area. In 1875, David Ferrier, working at King's College, in London, reported that monkeys were blind after removal of part of the parietal lobe called the 'angular gyrus'. Ferrier's monkeys would not reach out for or grasp objects placed in front of their eyes, and he concluded that the angular gyrus was the seat of vision.

The novelist C. P. Snow famously claimed that there are 'two cultures' – the scientific and the rest. For daring to include science in 'culture' at all, he was brutally attacked by the literary critic F. R. Levis, who found himself unable to acknowledge Snow's claims to being a novelist, but allowed him, amongst other things, the uttering of 'panoptic pseudo-cogences'. However, literary critics have no monopoly on nastiness: scientists can be just as gleefully vicious when they get the chance, and cannot resist the pleasure of exposing a rival's mistake. It is not enough to succeed: others must fail! Ferrier's theory of the angular gyrus was savagely attacked by the German physiologist Munk (1881), who held the view (now accepted) that the visual cortex is located in the occipital lobe at the back of the head. Working in the

Berlin Veterinary School, Professor Munk found that removal of the occipital lobe on one side made the monkey completely blind on the opposite side of space. Munk was not impressed by Ferrier's counter-suggestion that the occipital lobe was the seat of hunger, and declined initially to say anything about Ferrier's work, 'because there was nothing good to say about it'. Later he abandoned this benevolent silence and thundered that Ferrier's observations 'are worthless and gratuitous constructions since the operated animals were examined by Mr Ferrier in quite an insufficient manner and only at the time of general depression of brain function' – in other words, just after the operation. This was hard to avoid, since the animals generally succumbed to post-operative infection, but at the same time that Ferrier was carrying out his experiments on monkeys, his surgical colleague Lister was revolutionising surgery by introducing sterile techniques. His 'Puffing Billy' spread a fine mist of carbolic around the operating theatre, and dispelled the mists of ignorance that had doomed so many patients to death from post-operative infections. Ferrier profited from these advances to study his monkeys for longer periods of time after the operation, and it soon became clear even to him that the complete blindness he had described was temporary. The defects that remained were much milder, but nonetheless significant: it seemed that the defect was in the visual guidance of movement: 'On the fourth day there was some indication of returning vision. A piece of orange was held before it, whereupon it came forward in a groping manner and tried to lay hold but missed repeatedly. When a piece of orange was laid on the floor it stretched out its hand over it, short of it, and round about it before it succeeded in securing it.'

It did not take long to find similar problems in our own species. Bálint, in 1909, described a patient who had problems in reaching out for objects with his right hand. The patient (who had damage to the parietal lobes on both sides of the brain) was described as having optic ataxia ('ataxia' means 'without movement'), and also had problems in moving his eyes voluntarily. The neurologist Gordon Holmes concluded that patients with optic ataxia have a difficulty in localising an object in space in relation to their own body: in other words, they have a 'frame of reference' problem.

When we reach out to grasp an object, the brain needs to to know the spatial positions of both the hand and the object. These could be described in a number of ways. For example, if we can see both our hand and the object, their positions could be described in an 'eye-centred' frame of reference. As its name suggests, a frame of reference is a system for describing the position of objects in a fixed framework, like latitude and longitude for objects on the Earth's surface. An equivalent 'polar frame' describes the position of an object by its longitude and distance from the North Pole. In a frame of reference, the 'origin' (for example, the position of the zero line of longitude) is evidently arbitrary. An international conference in 1911 recognised the Greenwich Meridian as the zero line of longitude, and therefore made Greenwich the centre of the frame. Earlier, however, the French had their own reference frame, centred (naturally enough) in Paris. The Paris Meridian was the brainchild of the Abbé Picard, born in 1620 at La Flèche, in Anjou, and a founder member of the Académie des Sciences. On the day of the summer solstice in 1667 the observatory of Paris was opened in Faubourg St Jacques, in those days far enough from the centre of Paris to avoid light pollution, and the great North–South circle running through the observatory and the poles became the official Paris Meridian of zero longitude.

The supremacy of the Greenwich Meridian was decided in the end by British sea power; but if both the French and the British systems had remained in operation, there would have been two sets of maps, with zero longitude in different positions – an inconvenience, like having to add an hour to one's watch when travelling from London to Paris, but not a major one, since to translate between the two all we have to do is to subtract (or add) the difference in longitude between London and Paris. This simple bit of arithmetic is an example of a translation between frames of reference or, as mathematicians prefer to say, 'a transformation of coordinates'.

The problem of transforming frames of reference between different observers led the young Albert Einstein to his theory of relativity. Translation between frames of reference is also at the heart of the problem of representing space in the brain. Our intuition tells us that there is a single space in which we see objects, sense their positions around us with our eyes shut, and reach out to grasp them. This amounts to saying that there is a single frame of reference for all the activities that demand the use of space; but new evidence suggests that there are many different frames of reference in the brain and thus many spaces: 'The traditional view of the representation of space, supported by subjective experience, is that we construct a single spatial map of the world in which objects and actions are represented in a unitary framework. The alternative view holds that the brain constructs multiple spatial representations with each representation linked to a different action or region of space' (Colby and Goldberg).

This idea may turn out to be the most important idea about space since Einstein imagined himself sitting himself on a beam of light.

The simplest frame of reference for visual space is the eye itself. When we look directly at an object in front of us, its image falls on the region of the retina called the fovea, where we have our highest acuity. In the periphery of our vision is a chair, to which we now direct our attention. The position of the image of the chair on the retina can be described by its distance and angle from the fovea: a 'vector', which tells us how to move our eyes to the chair. We start out with a vector specifying the angle and distance of the target from the fovea and move our eyes until the distance or 'error signal' is zero. A similar trick could be used to move our hand towards a target if we can see both hand and target. Primates nearly always move their eyes towards a target if they are thinking of reaching out to grasp it. This means that the vector joining the hand (in the retinal frame) to the fovea is also a vector for moving the hand. Since the brain uses this efficient mechanism to move the eyes, it would be surprising if it did not use it as a crib for the visually controlled pointing of the arm. Indeed, experiments have shown that an eye movement to a target is speeded up if we simultaneously reach for that target with the hand.

We can get a long way with an eye-centred map, but this does not mean that the map is located literally in the eye. For a start, we have two eyes, which are eventually combined into a single map. Another problem with having the map in the eye is that we should forget the visual position of objects in space as soon as we closed our eyes. The retina has a memory measured in hundredths of a second, but simple experiments show that we can remember the positions of objects in the dark for tens of seconds, even if we move our eyes about during the memory period. Let the eyes roam around a room or landscape containing a number of objects, such as teacups or trees. One of these objects is selected as a target, and the eyes are moved to look in its direction. The eyes are then firmly shut, and are moved around behind the closed eyelids, while a mental image of the target is maintained. The mental image of the target stays roughly in the same place, in spite of the eye movements. After 5 seconds or so, with the eyes still shut, the arm is pointed firmly with the index finger extended towards the remembered direction of the target. Although this pointing is done literally in the dark, the pointing movement is surprisingly accurate, as may be seen by opening the eyes and looking along the line of the extended arm and finger towards the target. Of course, the pointing is not completely accurate, and the further away the final position of the eye from its position when pointing at the target, the larger the error is likely to be. Also, if instead of merely pointing at the target we try to grasp it (assuming it to be within reach), the error in the third dimension of distance is greater than the error in angle. However, as Dr Johnson observed of a dog walking on its hind legs, the surprising thing is that the performance is possible at all.

The crude explanation is obvious: we retain some sort of mental image of the object's position in space. We can point at this mental image just as we can point at a real target in space; but where is the space in which the mental image is located? How is the position of an object defined within it, and how is this position finally translated into a set of commands to move the arm? Why does the remembered position of the target in space not move when we move our eyes? Most likely the eye-centred frame is not in the retina itself, but in some part of the brain that represents the world with the fovea at its centre. This internal map can remember the visual directions of objects relative to the fovea, including the arm. It can also track the movements of the eye, and of the hand, even in the dark. The problem of tracking an object in the dark is similar to that of navigating a boat that has entered a dense bank of fog (before the days of GPS). One method is to keep track of the boat's speed and heading and use this information to update current position (dead reckoning). In the case of the arm, dead reckoning would correspond to keeping a record of the sequence of commands issued from the brain to move the arm. Physiologists since Helmholtz have called this record an 'efference copy'. It may seem an odd idea that we know where we are because we keep an accurate record of our own movement commands, but as the physiologist Pat Merton pithily remarked, '... there is no reason why we should not be able to judge the size of the motor volleys leaving the brain as accurately as we judge the size of the sensory volleys arriving.' In other words, our brain knows as much about its own movements through space as it does about the world outside.

If we could look at the 'eye-centred map' from outside the brain, it would resemble a giant operations board, in which grid lines represent the retina, and various tokens represent outside objects and the parts of our own body. Every time the eyes move, the positions of all the tokens except one move within it, but maintain the same relations to one another. The exception is the token marked 'fovea', which always stays in the middle of the map. Could such a 'dynamic map', as it has been called, be the physical basis for our experience of visual direction? An obvious objection is that the world does not move when we move our eyes. The reasons for this 'stability of the visual world' have been much debated, not least in the context of reading, first studied by Emile Javal.

Javal was born in 1839, the son of a Jewish banker, and worked at the University of Paris, where he followed the admirable French tradition of providing practical care for the deaf and blind, a tradition started after the revolution of 1789 by the Abbé de l'Epée, inventor of the first lip-reading system. Javal wanted to cure squint and is sometimes called the Father of Orthoptists. Sadly, he became completely blind himself in 1900, but reacted typically by writing a book of practical advice for others in the same predicament. He had another, more curious, claim to fame, as we can read in a contemporary obituary: 'La plimulto de ni konis la mortinton kiel eminenten blinden esperantiston.'

Javal was a founder Esperantist; but luckily he published his work on eye movements in French. Amongst other things, he observed that the eye movements of people reading text are not smooth, as they seem to be to the person making them, but jerky. The eyes rest on one word for a few tenths of a second, and then jump abruptly to another place in the text. No matter how hard we may try to move our eyes smoothly across the page they always move in spasms. These jerky movements are called 'saccades', after an old French word for the movement of a cart with square wheels. Why do we fail to perceive these abrupt displacements of the text on the retina when we are reading?

The American physiologist Dodge followed up Javal's observations with some elegant experiments. He first noted that his own eye movements were invisible to him in a mirror. Perhaps the displacements of the eye are too small to be perceived? This can be ruled out by watching the eyes of another person in a mirror. The very movements that are invisible to the person making them are clearly visible to the bystander – a striking proof of the difference between looking at the eyes and looking through them. Another of Dodge's experiments – easily repeated – uses two pieces of cardboard and some pieces of coloured paper. Two thin vertical slits are cut in each of the cards, which are then positioned one behind the other and in front of one eye so that we can see through both the slits only when the eye is pointing straight ahead. The observer then looks to the right of the nearer slit so that the further slit is invisible. A piece of coloured paper is placed behind the further slit, without telling the observer its colour. The observer then makes a rapid voluntary eye movement to a point left-wards of the slit. What is the colour of the paper behind the further slit? Observers are not able to tell; yet during the eye movement there must have been an instant when the images of the slits lined up and the colour was present on the retina. Apparently, the sensation was censored or suppressed, explaining (according to Dodge) why we do not see the world moving when we move our eye.

Against this, it could (and has been) argued that the colour in Dodge's experiment was too briefly presented to be perceived, or that it was too blurred by its rapid passage over the retina, rather than being actively censored by the brain. Colour is actually rather a bad choice of sensation for the experiment, since the mechanisms for colour perception are now known to be very sluggish, and take time to register in con-sciousness. We are not, in fact, totally blind during our eye movements. If we look out of the window of a train and make a rapid eye movement in the opposite direction to the train's motion while looking at the track, we can sometimes see an unblurred image of the sleepers. The eye movement counteracts the rapid movement of the track caused by motion of the train and momentarily stabilises the image on the retina, allowing it to be seen. This would not happen if perception were censored during an eye movement. Laboratory experiments show that objects presented briefly during eye movements are harder, but not impossible, to see. The evidence may seem confusing at first, but there is a solution. Perhaps when we make an eye movement, the spatial map goes 'off line' for a short time while the positions of objects in the eye-centred map are adjusted. These positional adjustments in the map are invisible to us. However, this would not prevent objects flashed during the saccade from becoming visible *afterwards*, even if their position in the map were somewhat distorted. Laboratory experiments have demonstrated this spatial distortion, and have even shown that it starts in time slightly before the eye movement takes place.

Another experiment shows what happens when the updating mech-anism fails. Slight pressure against the lower eyelid (not the eye!) with a finger or cotton-wool pad moves the eye in its orbit. Now the world really does seem to move. Apparently the instruction to move the eye with the hand does not get through to the mechanism that suppresses movement signals. Here is another experiment: touch an object with the index finger of the hand, move the hand behind the back, and then displace the eye in its orbit with the finger of the other hand. Immediately try to touch the object again with the hand, moving it rapidly from behind the back. There is a large error in the pointing, as if the hand has taken no account of the displacement of the image on the retina. The idea of a dynamic map in an eye-centred frame can explain this phenomenon. When the eye is moved in this unusual way, there is no signal to cause updating of the position of remembered objects in the reference frame; but the position of the images of the objects on the retina does change, so they are experienced as changing position. The hand, however, is invisible behind the back, so its position in the frame is unaltered; this changes its position relative to the perceived position of the target, with the result that we make an error in reaching. The error very rapidly disappears as we make further movements, because the position of the hand in the reference frame is altered when we see it.

A few simple experiments have taken us quite a long way towards understanding the complex transformations that happen to our spatial map when we move our eyes; but to go further we need more accurate measurements. Several recent experiments have supported the idea of a dynamic, eye-centred map. One experiment measured exactly how accurately the hand can be moved to a briefly flashed target in the dark. If the target is flashed in a straight-ahead position, so that its image falls in the centre of the eye, reaching is highly accurate. However, if the observer is looking to the left of centre when the target is flashed, so that it falls in the peripheral part of the retina, the following hand movement shows a systematic error: the hand is moved to the right of the midline. This tells us that there is an error in placing the target in the eye-centred map. (Perhaps we overestimate the angle through which the eye has moved.) Suppose the observer now sees a brief flash of the target when looking straight ahead, and then moves the eye to a peripheral location *before* making the hand movement. The position of the target when it was first flashed is accurately registered in the frame because it was straight ahead. However, when the eye is moved, the target position is updated to its new, but erroneous, position. The observer should therefore make a pointing error exactly the same as if the target had been flashed in the periphery, and this is exactly what happens.

The experiment works with sounds as well as lights. A small loud-speaker dead ahead of the observer emitted bursts of noise, which the observer tried to point towards after a memory period during which they either kept their eyes straight ahead, or moved them to follow a pointer to a position 10 degrees from dead ahead. The results were the same as they had been for lights. Movement of the eyes rightwards during the delay interval caused the observers to point to the *left* of the loudspeaker. Exactly the same was found when observers tried to point to their right foot, which was extended (invisibly) in front of them, or even when observers simply tried to point to the imagined position dead ahead of them. These experiments tell us that the positions of remembered lights, sounds and even limb positions are registered in a retinal reference frame.

In another experiment, using 'virtual reality', observers saw a three-dimensional virtual world, or 'workspace', in which they could move their arm. They could not see their arm directly, but were shown the location of their pointing finger as a small green cube, which moved about as they moved their real arm in the virtual workspace. Once the observer was familiar with the set-up, the position of the virtual finger was altered, so that when the observer tried to point, it appeared to them that they made an error. This is exactly like placing a prism in front of the eye, except that the distortion applied to one small part of space only. Given practice reaching to this part of space alone, the observers rapidly adapted, as they do in prism experiments. We know from the prism experiments that the explanation of the adaptation is that the observer has shifted the position of the hand in a visual reference frame. But where is that reference frame centred? The traditional prism experiment does not answer this question, but the virtual-reality experiment went on to see how the observer reached to targets in other parts of space, where they had not previously experienced the distortion. The pattern of new reaching errors betrayed the nature of the map: it is a spherical map, like that of a three-dimensional globe, centred between the eyes. Young children are wiser than they know when they locate 'me' between the eyes.

The parietal lobe is strategically placed to translate vision into action. It receives input from Munk's visual cortex V1, which provides information in an eye-centred frame. The visual areas of the parietal lobe send tendrils to the superior colliculus, where they can influence eye movements. They also have a main-line pathway linking them to the second brain in our head: the enigmatic cerebellum. We think of our massive cerebral hemispheres as being the defining feature of our species (that is what our cerebrum thinks, at any rate), yet the cerebellum has increased in size fourfold in the last 10 million years, while the whole brain has increased only by three times. The cerebellum contains 15 million cells on its output side alone, and each of these can make up to 200,000 connections with other cells – more than any other nerve cell in the brain. Despite its vast size it is still difficult to say precisely what the cerebellum does. A hoary old myth relates that a Cambridge window cleaner was found on post mortem to lack a cerebellum entirely, but the brain cannot now be found. (The story belongs with another apocryphal story, of an *erratum* slip in the first Cambridge edition of the Table of Random Numbers.) Whatever the effects of being born without a cerebellum might be, damage to it in the adult definitely causes huge impairments in movement and posture. One of the main long-distance pathways in the brain connects the cerebellum to the parietal lobe.

Ferrier's monkeys had problems in reaching for objects, or moving their eyes towards them, like human patients with optic ataxia and parietal-lobe damage. Is the parietal lobe the location of the maps that transform the picture in the eye into the framework of action? One area of the parietal lobe, the lateral intraparietal area, or LIP, is a strong candidate for an eye-movement map. If a monkey is planning an eye movement from A to B, nerve cells in LIP begin to fire in a location corresponding to B, even before the movement is made. The map has an eye-centred reference frame – in other words, B is defined with respect to the centre of the retina. It is like the map in the deep layers of the superior colliculus, where nerve cells fire just before a movement is made in a map position corresponding to the position of the target on the retina. Electrical stimulation of these cells also causes a movement of the eye to the target location, even if the monkey had no intention to move. The eye-movement map in the colliculus is a well-understood analogue computer for translating retinal information into movement. What does the parietal lobe add to this already-clever mechanism?

The answer is 'memory and planning'. If a monkey is about to make an eye movement to a target, nerve cells in area LIP start firing in the map position corresponding to the target position, even before the movement is made. In other words, these cells normally respond to an object in the target position, but they are now responding to the intention to move the eyes there. The frame of reference for these anticipatory eye movements is based on the retina, but shows memory and remapping. If the monkey has to move its eyes from A to B to C, nerve cells in LIP fire in the map position corresponding to C. However, when the eye movement is made from A to B, this activity is transferred to a new set of cells, in the map position corresponding to the new visual direction of C, even though C is now invisible.

Remapping is not an entirely automatic process. It depends on the monkey's knowledge and experience, and does not happen if the monkey learns that the invisible object moves in the dark so as to keep the same position on the retina. Perhaps the monkey imagines the object moving in space, like Proust's narrator with his objects 'whirling madly through the darkness'. We can form vivid spatial images of objects moving in the dark and use these images to guide our actions. For example, if we move our finger to and fro in the dark and attend to its tip, our eyes pursue it as if it were really visible. Imagination can move the eyes, even in the light. If we look at the 'snow' on an out-of-tune TV screen, we can pursue a snowflake across the screen with our eyes, even though no actual 'flake' is present on the screen for more than a few millionths of a second.

LIP plans eye movements. What about reaching for an object with the hand? The problem here is to represent both the eye and the hand in a common space. This is difficult: the eye can move in the head, the head can move relative to the shoulder, and the hand can move relative to the shoulder. One idea is that the brain breaks down the problem into several stages. First, it takes account of head movement, by transferring retinal position into a head-centred frame. Then, because the head can move on the neck, the head-centred frame is transferred into a trunk-centred frame. Finally, because the hand can move relative to the shoulder, the frame is transferred into one that is arm- or hand-centred. This is a neat scheme, but is there any evidence that the brain does things this way? Unfortunately, the search for 'head-centred' maps in the parietal cortex and elsewhere has not found any: 'the great tragedy of Science – the slaying of a beautiful hypothesis by an ugly fact', as Thomas Henry Huxley put it in another context. However, what has been found is in some ways more interesting. Many retina-centred nerve cells, including some in area LIP, do not change their preferred position on the retina when the head or other part of the body moves, but they do change their rate of firing. Sets of neurones like these have been dubbed 'gain fields', on the grounds that the 'gain' or amplification of the signal is affected by body position. Since the head direction changes the firing rate in many nerve cells, not just one, it has been suggested that we have here an elaborate code, distributed over many nerve cells, for correcting head position.

There is an alternative explanation. A clue is that electrical stimulation of the superior colliculus, close to the actual eye-movement machinery, produces shifts of both eye and head. The superior colliculus was originally supposed to be a simple machine, which moved the eyes in a fixed direction and angle, no matter what the position of the eyes in the head – the so-called 'fixed vector' model. It would therefore be the responsibility of 'higher' areas of the brain to calculate what that vector should be, taking into account the position of the eyes in the head; but in fact the colliculus itself can make allowance for head position. The brain is apparently an inveterate procrastinator, hanging on to its retina-centred frame for eye movement until the last possible moment.

The arm may be another procrastinator. Another area of the posterior parietal cortex, known as the 'parietal reach region' (PRR), is involved in the planning of reaching movements. When a monkey is about to reach out and touch a target, nerve cells in the PRR begin to fire before the movement is made. Different nerve cells fire according to the position of the object in space. Once again, however, the question is whether position relative to the arm, or position on the retina, is more important. It appears to be the retina. If the arm is placed in different positions before the start of the reach, the preferred target position (in outside space) does not change – in other words, there is no remapping. But remapping does take place if the eyes move while the monkey is waiting to make the hand movement. Nerve cells in the PRR behave exactly like those in the eye-movement area LIP, except that they are involved in the planning of arm movements, not eye movements. In both cases the frame of reference is the retina. Transformation of the retina-based signal into the instruction to move the arm seems to take place 'downstream' of the parietal reach area, just like the instructions to move the eyes themselves.

We have assumed so far that vision provides the only information about the position of our arm in space. This is only part of the story. The joints and muscles also give us information – not very accurate information, to be sure, but better than none. Some nerve cells in the parietal lobe of the monkey change their rate of firing when the monkey's arm changes position, even if the arm is invisible beneath a table; but even these neurones do not escape the all-pervasive influence of vision. In a somewhat bizarre experiment, the services of a taxidermist were engaged to place a fake monkey limb in front of the animal, whose own arm was invisible. Nerve cells in area 5 of the parietal lobe

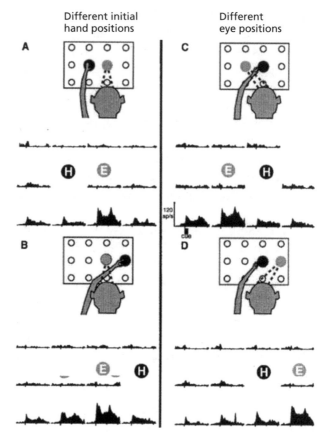

Figure 11.1 A nerve cell in the PRR of a monkey fires just before the monkey reaches out to touch a light that has flashed in the receptive field of the cell. The bar graphs show the response of the cell to a target in different spatial positions.

responded to movements of this fake limb as if it were the real arm. If a particular neurone favoured a position of the real arm to the left of the midline, it also favoured movement of the fake arm to the left. The two sources of information combined so that the neurone fired most vigorously when both the real (invisible) and fake arm coincided in space.

Sound also has to be put together with vision and touch. Sounds can be localised in space, because we have two ears. Sounds coming from the left side of space are slightly louder in the left ear than the right, and arrive in the left ear slightly earlier in time. Both these sources of information are used by the brain to localise sounds (hence the success of stereophonic headphones, which artificially reproduce these differences between the ears). In a classic experiment carried out at Bell Laboratories in New Jersey, observers wore a prism in front of their eyes to change the visual direction of objects on the retina. After they had adapted and could point to visible objects without error, they were asked to point to an invisible sound source. They pointed in the wrong direction, as if they had compensated for the direction of the sound as well as of the visual image. This could be simply explained by an adjustment of the arm-movement signal downstream of separate visual and auditory maps; but observations on owls show that the visual and auditory maps of space are intimately connected through experience. Owls localise their prey both by vision and by hearing. Like us, the owl has two ears, but to help it localise sounds even more accurately in the up–down plane the ear on one side is higher than on the other. There are separate visual and auditory maps in the owl's optic tectum (which we met previously in the frog). One map is activated by light, and the other by sound, but they are in precise registration, so that a light and a sound coming from the same direction activate neighbouring nerve cells in the two maps. Philosophers like Descartes who dismissed the importance of images in the brain would have considered this registration as a meaningless coincidence. They would have been wrong. If the young owl has prisms put before its eyes to shift the visual direction of objects, the visual and auditory maps are no longer in register. When the owl hears a sound it points its head towards it, but in the wrong direction to centre the image in its eye. After some experience, the error is corrected; and the auditory map in the tectum is found to have shifted also, to be once again in precise alignment with the visual map. In the analogue computer that is the brain, position matters.

The conclusion is that there are several maps of space in the brain. To begin with we have the relatively simple sensory maps in areas like the primary visual cortex (V1), which are little affected by whatever plans we might have to act on the basis of the information they provide. These maps tell us about the position of objects relative to our direction of gaze, nothing more. They are gradually transformed by the addition of information about eye and limb position into other maps, closer to the planning of movement. Some of these transformations take place in downstream structures like the colliculus, but they also happen in the multiple maps of the parietal lobe. The parietal lobe contains a bewildering variety of specialised maps, which seem set to continue their number with further research. As two authorities on the parietal lobe recently put it: 'The space around us is represented not once but many times in parietal cortex.' But we should not get carried away by the idea of thousands of maps with different reference frames. Keeping the maps in register is an important problem, and to a large degree the visual system solves this problem by the simple device of hanging on to an eye-centred frame of reference as long as possible. The visual direction of an object with respect to the centre of our eye is not just the most basic but also the most enduring frame of reference for vision, and even for other senses, such as hearing.

If there are visual maps all over the brain, it is natural to ask which of them are most important for our conscious experience of space. Is the map in the primary visual cortex conscious? What about the parietal lobe, or the optic tectum, for that matter? The next section examines the idea that only some areas of the brain are involved in our conscious experience. Readers should skip this section if they think that the relationship between philosophy and science is like that between pigeons and statues.

PART FOUR

THE LOCALISATION OF AWARENESS

12

Who Killed the Chauffeur?

In Raymond Chandler's novel *The Big Sleep* (1939), Owen Taylor is the chauffeur for the Sternwood family. Early in the book he is found dead at the wheel of one of the Sternwood cars in the surf off Lido fish pier. Private Investigator Philip Marlowe is present as the police and the medical examiner argue about whether Taylor's death is murder or suicide. The ME thinks he was blackjacked before hitting the water. Ten years after publication of *The Big Sleep*, Chandler wrote from La Jolla to his publisher Hamish Hamilton:

> I remember several years ago when Howard Hawks was making *The Big Sleep*, the movie, he and Bogart got into an argument as to whether one of the characters was murdered or committed suicide. They sent me a wire (there's a joke about this too) asking me, and dammit I didn't know either. Of course I got hooted at. The joke was in connection with Jack Warner, the head of Warner Bros. Believe it or not he saw the wire, the wire cost the studio seventy cents, and he called Hawks up and asked him whether it was really necessary to send a telegram about a point like that.

The point of all this nonsense is that hardly anyone spots the loose end in the plot. No one but an English exponent of the 'gentle art of murder' would come out of the film saying, 'But who killed the chauffeur?' Jack Warner was right about the seventy cents, and Sam Goldwyn was right about movies: motion pictures are for entertainment; messages should be delivered by Western Union.

The failure of most readers to spot problems like Taylor's death could be put down to the complexity of plot and the fallibility of memory; but other errors in films happen over a much shorter time-scale. In Orson Welles' masterpiece *Citizen Kane* the scene in which

Kane's wife is leaving him shows an open suitcase; the next shot, supposedly seconds later, shows the same suitcase closed. The function of continuity checks in movies is to prevent these things happening. Much of this effort is wasted. Audiences are, in fact, oblivious even to quite dramatic failures in continuity. The classic 1944 film noir version of Chandler's novel *Farewell my Lovely* (*Murder my Sweet* in the US), starring Dick Powell, has a tense scene between Philip Marlowe and Moose Molloy in a room where they are lit by a flashing neon sign outside the window. Director Dmytryk had to face insuperable problems in matching the different cuts across the on–off cycle of the light. Even in the final edited version the flashing stutters, in a way that would be instantly apparent in a sound track. Audiences did not notice, however, even though they must have been looking at the faces of the actors; apparently even film students miss the error. Inevitably, there are whole Web sites devoted to cataloguing errors in films. From them we learn about some colossally uninteresting continuity errors in recent films such as *Silence of the Lambs*, as well as errors of fact. (Did you know that Clarice could not possibly have the degree she claimed from the University of Virginia?) None of these errors matters. You have to be a geek to find them, and even worse to put them on a Web site. Anachronisms such as a wristwatch on Julius Caesar are similarly hard to spot – unless we pay attention.

Continuity blindness tells us that we take in less from our eyes than we think. It is tempting, but wrong, to think of our visual image as like a detailed photograph. The visual image *appears* to be a plenitude, with a lightness value at every point; but is it? If there is a large patch of uniform green in the image, there would be little point in describing it point by point. This would amount to coding it in Pixelese, and Pixelese is a deeply redundant language. 'Switching off' is a common response to redundancy. If, like the writer, you live in a voting constituency where the vast majority of your neighbours would vote for a hamster provided it wore a red rosette, your own vote is a waste of time. You save energy by staying at home. On the other hand, if you live in a marginal constituency, where you cannot predict the votes of your neighbours, your voice becomes important. Our visual brain uses the same logic, as we see in a computer-processed face image (see figure 12.1).

The image seems to be composed of uniform regions of different brightness. In fact, the image has been processed digitally to make most points in the image have the same lightness values. The interior points

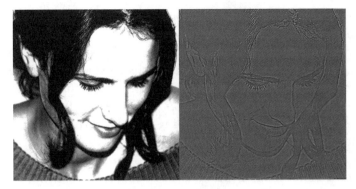

Figure 12.1 A face image processed to be a uniform grey except for ridges in its landscape

of the face and the hair have the same physical lightness values, as may be seen by using a small hole cut from a sheet of paper to examine them individually. The digital rule used to construct the image is similar to the one used in the retina and the primary visual cortex. If a pixel is surrounded by other points with the same initial lightness value, it is set to grey. If it is surrounded by darker points, it is set to white; if it is surrounded by lighter points, is it set to black. This highlights the boundaries between objects, but makes their interiors all the same. However, to our eye, the grey areas within objects seem different, according to the contrast at the border. Apparently, lightness values in the silent areas are 'filled in' at some higher level of visual processing.

'Filling in' also happens at the 'blind spot' – the place in the retina where the optic nerve fibres exit, and where there are no rods or cones. To see the blind spot, take a blank sheet of white paper and draw a small spot in the centre; then a cross two inches to the left. Close the right eye, and look steadily through the left eye at the paper held about one hand's length away from the eye, and note the appearance of the cross. As the paper is moved slowly away from or towards the eye, there should be a position at which the cross completely disappears. It has fallen in the blind spot.

Charles II is said to have decapitated tiresome dinner guests by placing them in his blind spot. If you want to try a similar trick, remember that one eye must be shut. The blind spots in the two eyes are in different places, and cover for one another. In spite of this, we are not ordinarily conscious of a gap in the visual image when we close one eye. Is this because we fill it in with some internal paint pot – or, more simply, that we ignore it? The idea behind the 'paint-pot' theory is that activity spreads from nerve cells outside the blind spot to stimulate the nerve cells inside; but isn't this rather like keeping a dog and doing one's own barking? First we have an energy-saving mechanism that reduces redundancy; then we waste the energy all over again by 'filling in'. The paint-pot theory makes sense only if the filling in happens at some higher level than the primary visual cortex, where rather small numbers of nerve cells are involved. If this is so, the argument between 'inattentive filling in' and 'active filling in' may turn out to be mainly semantic.

The map in the primary visual cortex covers the whole of our visual field, with a large magnification of the central part. When we attend to one part of the visual field we nearly always move our eyes there, so that it is represented in the region of clearest vision; but what happens to the rest of the map when we are attending to the centre? Common experience suggests that the whole of the field remains visible, like a picture before our eyes, no matter how attentively we stare at the centre. After all, we can see the cat on the rug even if we are not looking directly at it; but to do so, it could be argued, we have to attend to the place where the cat is sitting. Perhaps we had no conscious awareness of the cat until we moved our attention there. We could try to demonstrate this by asking an observer to describe a scene after closing their eyes. They might fail to mention the cat; but does this prove that they never saw it? They might have seen it and forgotten. In 'Kim's game', the contestant is shown a tray containing a number of objects, such as a knife, a book and a set of keys. After the tray is removed they are asked to name the objects. Many objects are forgotten, despite frantic efforts to put them into memory. Plainly, we do not imprint a photograph of the scene in our mind for more than a fraction of a second, if ever.

It may seem an odd idea – unprovable even – that most perceptions disappear immediately without trace; but everyday experience suggests that we can be aware of our surroundings even if we have little or no memory. If we are driving a car along a habitual route and thinking about work, we might be quite incapable, if challenged, of saying how many cars we had overtaken in the last ten minutes. Some psychologists would infer from this that we were literally unconscious of what was happening on the road, but this is implausible. If driving does not need 'care and attention', it is a bit hard to know why there is a legal offence in England and Wales of driving without it. It would be no defence against a charge of dangerous driving to say, 'I was thinking about work, and not attending to what was going on.'

A common trick used on television or in the movies to get the viewer's attention is to present a rapid series of images one on top of the other – click-click-click – too quickly for us to say what they were. We may not be able to say what they were, but there is the irritating impression just the same that we *saw* them. The impression is different from the one seen when the frames are presented so rapidly that they fuse into a blur. We feel that we see each image – the tiger, for example – individually, but too briefly to fix it into verbal memory. Of course, this could all be an illusion or hallucination, and we never really saw the images at all, or saw them in such poor detail that we could not distinguish individuals; but in this case, why do we not hallucinate the faces when they are presented too rapidly; and why, if asked immediately after the movie 'Was there a tiger?', can we say 'Yes'?

The challenge for psychologists, then, is to design experiments that distinguish between immediate perception and memory. One such is based on the proposition that it is hard to do two things at the same time – chew gum and walk straight, for instance. If we carry out a demanding task like watching a rapid sequence of photographs and pressing a button whenever a dog appears, we are less accurate at some 'secondary task' in a different place on the screen. We may even miss quite large changes in the unattended area completely, such as the gradual change in the colour of a car from red to blue. One way of getting the observer's attention is to get them to press a button whenever the letter 'G' occurs in a string of letters – easy enough, one might think, but the letters are presented on top of one another at a rate of several per second. There is little time left over to decide whether another letter, presented in the periphery of the visual field, is in 10 point or 14 point type. Interestingly, if the observer correctly intercepts a 'G' in the letter string, and is in the process of pressing the button, she will often fail completely to note that another 'G' has occurred. This has been called the 'attentional blink', the idea being that we are effectively blind for a short time during each detection. The implications are interesting. It cannot be the process of recognising a letter in itself that produces the blink, for there is no blink to an 'R' or indeed to any other letter but the target 'G'. It seems to be the decision to press the button that causes the mischief. Here we have more than a hint that attention and voluntary action are not separate but are the warp and woof of perception.

Another line of evidence that we see far less than we think we do is a popular variant of Kim's game in comics and magazines. We see two almost identical cartoons side by side and are invited to spot the seven differences. (There is a button missing from the clown's coat in the right-hand picture, for example.) The task is very hard, and to solve it we have to resort to manoeuvres such as counting the number of buttons on the coat. Try as we might to form a mental image of the first picture and compare it to the second, we fail. As soon as we have seen the difference it becomes obvious. This seems to mean that we never formed a mental image of the first picture at all. Our feeling that we have a mental image is self-deception. What we have is internal descriptions of the picture, not images, and these descriptions depend on attention to detail. The other possibility is that there is an image, which is so fugitive that it has gone by the time we move our eyes to the second picture. Finally, it could be that images exist, but we are unable to compare them. To decide which of these is true, psychologists have named the phenomenon 'change blindness' and experimented on it with interesting (and occasionally hilarious) results.

The first point to be made about change blindness is that it is easily overcome by a simple trick. If we flash the two images in succession like two frames of a movie, instead of looking at them side by side, the changes immediately 'pop out'. Either the changed features appear to move, or they flicker. This discovery dates back to the early motion-picture toy, the phenakistoscope, in which a rapidly rotating card reveals a parrot jumping in and out of his cage. Clearly we can compare the two images on either side of the card if they follow one another quickly in time on the same part of the eye. It follows logically that there must be some form of storage for each image over time. The principle of the phenakistoscope was exploited by astronomers with an instrument called the 'blink microscope' to find planets or comets that had moved against the background of the fixed stars. Two photographs taken at the same sidereal time were flashed in rapid sequence, and anything that had moved between the two 'popped out', even if the movement was as little as one-thousandth of the Moon's diameter. This, though, does not prove that we store a conscious visual image of every star in the photographs. Specialised movement detectors can do the job, or detectors of flicker on the eye. In other words, movement can be detected by low-level mechanisms, at a stage long before conscious recognition of objects. The same can be said about the other trick for overcoming change blindness: placing the two pictures in a stereoscope and noting features that do not match between the two eyes by their changes in depth. Astronomers did this with the 'stereocomparator'.

Breaking change blindness with a stereocomparator does not imply that the left and right eyes form separate mental images, which we then compare. Stereoscopic vision is accomplished by special-purpose analogue computers called 'binocular' nerve cells that have receptive fields at different places in the two eyes.

Another kind of fugitive visual image is not so easy to explain away by motion or stereo mechanisms. In classic experiments at Bell Laboratories in New Jersey, observers saw a very briefly flashed array of numbers and were asked to report what they had seen. They could report at most only two or three of the digits. If they were 'cued' beforehand to look at the digit in one position on the screen, they would always get it right. This supports the view that attention is required to put a visual impression into memory. However, the next result was the real surprise: observers could report a cued number even if the cue was presented several tenths of a second *after* the numbers were flashed up. Conclusion: there must be some short-term visual image, or 'icon', that lasts for a few tenths of a second after the flash of a single movie frame, and which contains full visual detail. But are we conscious of the details in the image for the short period during which it lasts? This is the hundred thousand dollar question, which is so hard to solve without looking into the brain itself. Storage of the icon might take place at some very early stage in the visual pathway – perhaps even in the retina – long before we become aware of it.

The icon can be completely abolished by a bright flash of light in the time interval between the presentation of the numbers and the cue. It is as if the flash wipes the slate clean and prevents the observer from reading the cued number. The same method has been used to wipe the slate clean in change-blindness experiments. The two pictures are shown in succession like a movie, but with a bright flash between them to destroy the icon. When this is done, the observer is unaware of large changes between the two images – for example, the disappearance of a jet engine from an aircraft wing. In Alfred Hitchcock's film *Rear Window*, James Stewart becomes convinced that his neighbour in a flat opposite has dismembered his wife and buried a body part in the flower bed below. He compares how the flower bed looks now with a colour slide taken a few weeks previously, and notices that the flowers are now shorter. Hitchcock illustrates the change by showing us the two images in succession. The change is totally invisible. It is unclear whether this is one of Hitchcock's jokes, or an unusual mistake about human perception.

Of course, if the change is sufficiently dramatic, it will be seen – images of the Manhattan skyline before and after 11 September would quickly tell their story; but this only reinforces the point that our attention has to be drawn to the part of the scene that has been changed, before we can spot what is different.

Psychologists have turned into magicians to demonstrate 'change blindness' on the street. An actor stops an innocent passer-by to ask for some directions. Two other actors walk between them carrying a screen that temporally obstructs the communication. Yet another actor hidden behind the screen changes places with the first. The substitution often goes unnoticed. Only if the change is sufficiently dramatic – a man for a woman, for example – does the observer do a 'double take'. An assistant in a record store dips down behind the counter to pick something up from the floor. A different person, hidden behind the counter, emerges. The substitution is often unnoticed by the customer.

Change blindness and the attentional blink are dramatic and entertaining phenomena, but they have not really solved the awkward question of how much we see in the first place, against how much we remember. Terms such as 'seeing' and 'remembering' are vague, and leave too much room for semantic argument. A more direct approach is to look inside the brain itself. Functional magnetic resonance imaging (fMRI for short) exploits the fact that the brain uses a lot of energy to send messages through its intricate circuits. The brain is only 2 per cent of the body mass, but during an average day it gobbles up 20 per cent of our calories, even if the intellect is suspended by watching television. Most of this energy is taken up by the complicated chemical machinery needed to pass nerve impulses between cells. When nerve cells are not firing, they need less energy, and this may be the reason – from the perspective of natural selection – why most nerve cells are silent most of the time. If all the nerve cells in our brain were active all of the time, we should all need to be bald to dissipate the heat. However, the little grey cells spring into action only when their particular contribution to perception, thought or action is needed; and when this happens, they withdraw oxygen from the tiny blood vessels from which they are never far distant. This BOLD (blood oxygen level depletion) response can be detected by perturbations of a powerful magnetic field in the fMRI machine. By computer-assisted analysis a three-dimensional map of the brain can be built up in which the oxygen-gobbling areas are shown as 'hot spots'.

Attention was memorably compared by the French philosopher

Maurice Merleau-Ponty to a searchlight, picking out its targets from a surrounding gloom. Searchlights use a lot of energy. If we take the searchlight metaphor literally, we expect nerve cells to increase their activity to an attended target, just as if the target were more strongly lit. In an fMRI experiment on change blindness, observers had to decide whether strings of rapidly flashed letters such as 'NZQ' followed by 'XBV' did or did not contain the letter 'X'. This was the 'primary task' meant to occupy their attention more or less fully. At the same time as the letters, faces were flashed up on a different part of the screen. Twice a second the faces disappeared and were replaced with either the same face or a different one. After this had happened twice, the observers were asked whether the faces were changed or not. The difficulty of the primary task was adjusted so that the observers spotted the face change on only half the trials. On the other trials they were 'blind' to the change. This, of course, could have been because they forgot the faces rather than being blind to them; but the advantage of functional imaging over verbal report is that we can look at what happened at the time the face was presented, rather than waiting for the observer to tell us what they have seen.

Results seemed to support the searchlight theory. A region called the 'fusiform face area' was more active when the change in face was seen than when it was missed by the observer. In a control task, where the images were of outdoor scenes rather than faces, there was no difference in the 'face area'. This seems to tell us that the searchlight is not in the primary visual cortex, but in 'higher' areas, such as those specialised for face recognition. However, the beautiful coloured maps we see in fMRI experiments have to be treated with some caution. They are not a direct vision of the brain in action, but more like supposed 'pictures' of the Universe 5 seconds after it was created, highly stylised and interpreted by a computer from slender data. Suppose we had a map of Britain showing the local increases in numbers of Alzheimer's cases between 1950 and 2002, colour coded for the statistical significance of the increase – in other words, regions where we could be very sure an increase had occurred would be coloured red, and regions where we were much less sure would be coloured blue. Such a map might very well show the cities in red and the Highlands of Scotland blue, not because there is any real difference in Alzheimer's between these regions, but because there are more people in cities, and therefore more cases. The more cases there are, the easier it is to be sure that an increase is a real one. To be meaningful the map would have to be divided up into regions that contained equal numbers of people. Applying this to the example of the face area, the problem is that the BOLD response in the face area is (by definition) greater to faces than to non-faces. It may be easier to find a statistically significant reduction in this response when it is large rather than small, and thus when faces are present rather than absent.

Another more direct way of looking for the 'searchlight' is to record from single cells in monkeys when they are attending to a target. At least we now know what the nerve cells are doing. There is little convincing evidence for a 'searchlight' in primary visual cortex V1; cells there respond to targets in much the same way irrespective of whether the monkey is attending to them. In the other V areas, attention does change the response of cells to a target. In V4, one experiment showed that attention was equivalent to a roughly 50 per cent increase in the strength of the target. Some increase in activity is even found when the monkey is attending inside the receptive field and there is no target within it; this has to be an effect of some 'top-down' process.

The 50 per cent increase in firing is a puzzle. How can it explain 'attention'? Suppose that there are two spots of light in our visual field, moving at right angles to one another and at different speeds. We are instructed to attend to whichever one we like, and then, when a buzzer sounds, to follow the attended spot with our eyes. According to the 'searchlight' theory, nerve cells responding to the attended target are responding a bit more vigorously than those responding to the unattended target, say, 50 per cent more strongly; but when we move our eyes we can only follow one of the targets. The movement cannot be 75 per cent to one target and 25 per cent to the other. Therefore, a choice has to be made between the nerve cells responding to the two targets, to decide which one of them will control the action. Now, if we can make this choice at the time we make the action, what is the purpose of the searchlight in the first place? Only if the searchlight totally switched off the activity of the unattended nerve cells would there be no choice to be made, and not even the most optimistic versions of the searchlight theory say that this is so. It cannot generally be the case that decisions always favour the more intense sensory input, or we should not be able to follow the dimmer of two moving spots with our eyes (which we can, easily).

Attention is about choosing between alternative courses of action. Sometimes these actions are external and observable, like moving the eyes. Sometimes they are internal, like tracking the spot 'in our mind's eye'. Theories of attention that concentrate on internal actions can be accused of straining at a gnat and swallowing a camel. By far the most obvious acts of attention are observable ones, such as moving our eyes to the person who is talking to us, or picking up one object from a clutter on the table. The idea that first we attend through some sort of searchlight, and then choose our course of action, may be fundamentally mistaken. The two processes are often the same. Recent electrical 'microstimulation' experiments on monkeys are suggesting as much. In these experiments, small electrical currents are applied to nerve cells in the brain to influence the animal's actions. In one experiment, stimulation was applied to a region of the frontal lobe known to produce eye movements – the 'frontal eye field'. Nerve cells there have 'motor fields' analogous to 'receptive fields' of sensory nerve cells. They are laid out in yet another map, where position corresponds to the region of space to which the monkey will move its eyes. In the experiment, the frontal eye field was stimulated at too low a strength to move the animal's eyes to a target in the visual field, but at a sufficient strength to make the animal move its attention there. The act of selecting an eye movement and the act of moving attention seem to depend on the same mechanism.

Another 'microstimulation' experiment shows that the decision to attend to an object can evoke a whole set of actions appropriate to that object. When we attend to a chair we see much more than an object with a horizontal platform and four legs. We see something we can sit on – unless we have a kind of 'object agnosia' where this ability is lost. A movie of someone sitting on a chair in the dark with lights attached to their joints produces an irresistible perception of a chair, despite the absence of any chair image. In the microstimulation experiment, monkeys were given the choice of tracking with their eyes either one of two targets moving in different directions and at different speeds. During the time while the monkey was making up its mind which target to track, microstimulation of the frontal eye field was applied to a motor field that would normally direct an eye movement to one of the two targets. This made the monkey 'make up its mind' to move its eyes to that target – not very surprising. What is surprising is that the instant the monkey's eye alighted on the selected target it started to pursue it with a further smooth eye movement at exactly the speed of that target, not the speed of the rejected target. Normally, it takes about a tenth of a second for the speed of pursuit to match that of the target, so the monkey must have chosen this tracking speed before it moved its eyes to the target. The implication is that the whole process of choosing which target to select, moving the eyes there, and pursuing it are all part of the same process.

The attractions of direct brain stimulation for localising awareness are obvious. Unfortunately, it is difficult to carry out in human beings, the only animals who can describe to us what they see. The next chapter describes the history of stimulating the conscious human brain directly with electromagnetic waves.

13

Where is Fancy Bred?

The history of electrical stimulation of the brain starts with the experiments of Benjamin Franklin in the eighteenth century. Early results were not exactly encouraging. A pullet given a powerful electric shock ran headlong against a wall, and 'on examination appeared perfectly blind'. A turkey of 10 lb weight was even less fortunate and was struck stone dead, but did 'eat uncommonly tender' (an argument not yet advanced by advocates of the electric chair, oddly enough). Communicating Franklin's experiments to the Royal Society of London, in 1751, William Watson, FRS cautioned members of his Club:

> Some times since it was imagined that deafness had been relieved by electrifying the patient, by drawing the snaps from his ears, and making him undergo the electrical commotion in the same manner (*sc* as the pullet). If hereafter this remedy should be fanatically applied to the eyes in this manner to restore the dimness of sight, I should not wonder, if perfect blindness were the consequence of the experiment.

Apparently, the idea of causing vision by direct electrical stimulation was already current (as it were). Weak shocks to the eyeball do indeed cause sensations of light, called 'phosphenes', similar to those seen when we press against the eyeball, or when the eye is struck a sudden blow. Of course, this does not mean that consciousness occurs in the retina, or in the optic nerve. Vision is possible without the eye. Patients who have lost their eyes, or had their optic nerves severed in an accident, can still have visual experiences in the form of hallucinations, dreams or vivid images. The Swiss naturalist Charles Bonnet (1720–83), whose main claim to fame is that he discovered parthenogenesis in aphids (and thought that it explained how single animals reproduced after the Biblical Flood), also gave his name to the Charles Bonnet syndrome, when he noticed that his grandfather, partially blinded by cataracts, hallucinated birds and buildings. Patients with the Charles Bonnet syndrome experience vivid hallucinations of faces, people or landscapes. The faces are often described as being ugly, with prominent eyes or teeth. Strange little people appear from nowhere, wearing hats or period costumes. They move in a realistic way. Since the patients with the syndrome have impaired vision from eye disease, their hallucinations are often more intense than their 'normal' perceptions. The obvious conclusion is that retinal images are not required for visual perceptions.

Even stronger evidence is that blind people can see small electrical pulses applied directly to the brain itself, which they experience as flashes of light, or 'phosphenes', with a particular location in space like stars in the night sky, depending on the part of the brain stimulated. Despite William Watson's dire warnings against 'fanatical' experiments, electrical stimulation is now being used to restore sight to blind people by linking the brain to a TV camera. A sixty-two-year-old patient who was totally blinded at the age of thirty-six, had an array of sixty-four electrodes – resembling silicon chips – implanted in his brain when he was forty-one years old. Stimulation of the array produces phosphenes covering an area of visual space roughly equal to a book held at arm's length. The array is connected via a computer to a small TV camera mounted on spectacle frames in front of the patient's right eye. The perceived location of phosphenes in space does not correspond in any simple way to the location of the electrodes in the array, and of course there is no third dimension (distance) in the image. A puzzling problem is that stimulation of a single electrode produces not one phosphene, but several with different locations in space. Perhaps the current is spreading to more than one brain area and, as we know, there are many different maps in the brain. Despite these multiple images, the patient can recognise eye-chart letters about 6 inches in size from a distance of 5 feet, and can count fingers on a hand held in front of his face. He travels alone in the New York metropolitan area and uses public transport, but it is not possible to say whether he uses his artificial vision to do this, since he was equally mobile before getting the implant.

There is a very long way to go before patients can be given an effective bionic eye. One problem is that the patient sees the TV image move whenever he moves his eyes. In normal vision, objects do not appear to move when we move our eyes, although their images on the retina do move. The explanation is that the brain takes the eye movement into account in perceiving the position of objects. When we put on magnifying spectacles for the first time, eye movements produce sickening lurches of the external world, because the amount of movement on the retina exceeds that expected from the eye movement. Strobe lights imprint a frozen image on our retina, which remains stationary when we move the eye, with equally nauseating results. The problem for the patient is that his eye movements do not move the TV camera, and therefore they seem to move the world. A simple linkage between the eye and a motorised camera should overcome this problem.

The astronauts on Apollo 11 experienced flashes of light with their eyes closed, and wondered if they were experiencing cosmic rays going through their heads. (Obviously, they had not been drinking alcohol, the usual explanation for this phenomenon.) A space-medicine expert called Toby Tobias checked this out by putting a black bag over his head and exposing himself to radiation in a cyclotron and, sure enough, he saw flashes. A less hazardous way of exposing the brain to electromagnetic radiation is to stimulate the brain by a very brief and intense magnetic pulse (Transcranial Magnetic Stimulation, or TMS for short). The magnetic field is confined to the area just under the stimulator, which means that it stimulates the nerve cells just under the electrode, and nowhere else (if the strength of the pulse is properly adjusted). Stimulation over the striate cortex produces flashes of lights in the visual direction expected from the anatomy. A man of sixty-one, blind for almost eight years through damage to his optic nerve, also sees phosphenes, but the mapping is not so precise as in the sighted observers, suggesting some loss of function. Phosphenes in normal observers obeyed Emmert's law, which states that the apparent size of an after-image on the retina increases if we look into the distance (see Appendix A, on 'Demonstrations'). Legend has it that an alcoholic psychologist observed Emmert's Law in his hallucinations of pink elephants. Phosphenes from TMS did the same.

TMS and electrically produced phosphenes tell us that activity in the occipital cortex leads to some forms of conscious experience, with or without the retina; but, of course, this does not prove that the experiences happen *in* the occipital cortex, any more than phosphenes from stimulation of the eye prove that perceptions happen in the retina. After all, perceptions can be produced by even cruder means, as Thomas

Hobbes knew in 1651: 'The cause of Sense is the Externall Body, or Object, which presseth the sense organ proper to each sense ... And as pressing, rubbing or striking the Eye, makes us fancy a light; and pressing the Eare, produceth a dinne, so do the bodies also we see, or hear, produce the same by their strong, though unobserved action' (Hobbes, *Leviathan*, 1651, chapter 1).

There is nothing magical about stimulation applied directly to the brain. Failure to understand this simple (but often missed) point led no less distinguished a figure than Jean-Paul Marat into error. Before starting his career as a popular agitator and journalist during the French Revolution, Marat led a shady existence as a medical man in England and Scotland, where he purchased an MD from the University of St Andrews in 1775. In his 'Philosophical Essay on Man' (1773), Marat considers the seat of sensation, starting with a succinct review of the possibilities: 'Anatomists agree, that we must look for the seat of the soul in the head; but they are not unanimous what place it occupies in that part of the body. Some place it in the *pineal gland*, others in the *corpus callosum*, others again in the *cerebrum*; some in the *cerebellum* and some in the *meninges*.'

There is scarcely less diversity of opinion amongst neuro-psychologists today, except that they would all reject the meninges – the membranes surrounding the brain. Unhappily, this is the one possibility Marat considers well founded. His evidence? First, he argued that brain-damaged soldiers can have large pieces of iron *inside* the brain, without experiencing any ill effects. There is, however, an even more convincing proof: thrust a scalpel into the meninges of a dog and it will 'vent the most doleful cries'; put the scalpel a good way into the substance of the brain and the animal will not give the least sign of any painful sensation.

The soldiers simply tell us that Marat was no more skilled in clinical observation than certain psychiatrists who thought that they could remove the frontal lobes of psychiatric patients without ill effects. As for the repellent experiments with doleful dogs, the real explanation is that the membranes, unlike the brain itself, contain pain receptors. Marat may or may not have been the same as the shadowy Le Maître of Warrington, who was suspected of stealing a gold medal from the Ashmolean Museum, in Oxford. What is certain, and documented in the painting by David (see plate section), is that he was fatally stabbed by Charlotte Corday in his bath – the only writer of a book on consciousness to have got his just deserts.

When we stimulate the striate cortex, the activity spreads to other areas of the occipital, temporal and parietal cortex, and eventually to the frontal lobe. Any or all of these areas may be necessary for perception to occur. Some may even be sufficient. Unravelling 'necessary and sufficient' causes in a complex, interconnected machine like the brain is similar to proving that carbon dioxide from power stations causes global warming – but a thousand times more difficult. For instance, the 'motion area' (V5) is arguably both necessary and sufficient for sensations of motion; 'necessary', because damage to it causes loss of sensitivity to motion in a human patient; 'sufficient', because single cells there mirror the perceptual abilities of conscious monkeys. However, V5 has connections 'forwards' to other areas, and even 'backwards' to the primary visual cortex. Perhaps V5 does not produce sensations unless V1 is active as well. One attempt to untie this Gordian knot examined the effect of TMS on the motion area in a patient without primary visual cortex. The patient (know by his initials, GY) is blind in the right half of space because of destruction of the primary visual cortex on the *left* side of the brain. In normal people, stimulation of V5 on one side of the brain produces motion-like sensations in the opposite side of space; but it did not do so in the blind half-field of GY, although he sometimes saw faint sensations in his *right* visual field. The reason why stimulation of V5 in normal observers causes sensation may be that this stimulation travels first from V5 to V1, and then back again in a form that causes sensation. The Gordian knot remains unravelled.

Can it be cut by colour? Again, brain damage gives us compelling evidence for a region or regions of the cerebral cortex necessary for normal perception. Inouye's patient Mr Tanaka confused reds, greens and blues, but could still name objects such as a cup. In the condition known as achromatopsia, colour sensation is lost but perception of motion and of black and white form survives. Achromatopsia is quite different from ordinary colour blindness, which is caused by missing or abnormal cones in the retina. The cones of the achromatopsic are normal, and she can see the boundary between two different colours just as well as a normal observer. What she cannot do is to name them: presumably she sees them as different shades of grey. The opposite condition is sometimes found in patients with carbon monoxide poisoning, who may retain the ability to name colours, but very little else. One patient (PB), who suffered lack of oxygen to the brain after an electric shock, still had conscious perception of colour, but was otherwise completely blind.

A further clue comes from 'colour synaesthetes' – people who experience colours when they hear or see words. A strong connection between sound and colour in the brain is suggested by the long history of attempts to build 'coloured organs', designed to play colours instead of sounds. In 1743 the Jesuit priest Bertrand Castel designed a stringed instrument combined with moving coloured tapes. In 1789 Charles Darwin's grandfather Erasmus suggested using coloured glass to project light from oil lamps in synchrony with music; the Darwin family can thus claim to have invented the discothèque. Another relative, Francis Galton, noted that the tendency of some people to experience colours in response to spoken words runs in families, but almost exclusively in the female line. Is 'synaesthesia' a genuine crossover of sensations from one modality to another? There are doubters, such as Professor Bianchi, a psychiatrist and Minister of Public Instruction in Italy in the 1900s, who supported the association theory: 'A servant of the author, like all the common people in Italy, used to call *turchino* (azure) *blu* (blue). Since then, the vowel *I* of the accented syllable of the word *turchino* has always made the author see *blu*, as *o* makes him see *rosso* (red) and *u nero* (black), vulgarly *nero-fumo* (soot).' In other words, synaesthesia is merely an example of 'associative learning', which makes us think 'dog' when we hear 'cat'.

Despite sceptics like Professor Bianchi, others think that synaesthetes have an unusual brain 'wiring diagram', which causes the 'colour area' to be activated by non-coloured words. A recent brain-imaging study examined a group of synaesthetes who experienced strong colours when they saw certain words or numbers. In the first part of the experiment synaesthetes and normal controls looked at coloured patterns while their brain activity was recorded. Compared to black–white patterns, coloured patterns caused greater activation in a small brain area V4, already suspected from the earlier work of Zeki of being a 'colour area'. This same area in the brains of the synaesthetes was also activated by 'coloured' words, but these words caused no significant activation in the same area of non-synaesthetes. Was this just 'associative learning', or was the wiring of the synaesthete brain unusual? To answer this, the non-synaesthetes were trained to associate words with colours by presenting them together. Even after they had learned the associations, the non-synaesthetes showed no activation of the colour area to spoken words; nor did efforts on their part to imagine colours. The experiment suggests that the brains of synae-sthetes are wired in an unusual way compared to 'normal' people, so that words activate brain areas that are normally activated during colour perception.

For many neuroscientists, fMRI finally cuts the Gordian knot. But perhaps we should remember the advice of a wise psychiatrist, asked by his colleagues what he thought of a new panacea: 'Use it quickly,' he said, 'before it stops working.' The basic idea of fMRI is that a brain area involved in perceiving colour (for example) will be more active when we are perceiving colour than when we are not. If this were true of the whole brain, we should have learned nothing. Therefore, it is just as important that there should be other areas that do *not* change their activity when we are perceiving colour; but does this mean that they are not involved in the perception of colour? Here we have to take account of a very significant limitation of fMRI as a technique for localising events in the brain: it does not measure the firing of nerve cells directly, but does so indirectly through the effect on the Blood Oxygen Level Depletion (BOLD) response – and the BOLD response is not very well localised, either in time or in space. At present, the spatial resolution of fMRI in the human brain is measured in millimetres, or hundreds of thousands of cells. Within an area of that size, quite different cells might be active during two different brain scans, without their being any difference as far as the BOLD response is concerned.

This is obviously true for the retina. Red squares and green squares cause different patterns of activity in long wavelength ('red') and medium wavelength ('green') cone receptors. With suitably placed elec-trodes we would be able to tell whether the person was looking at the red square or the green from the response of the retina; but this dif-ference would be completely undetectable with an instrument having the same poor spatial resolving power as the BOLD response. We can take this argument even further into the brain. The BOLD response in V1 does not significantly differ for coloured and black–white stimuli; yet we know from experiments on single nerve cells in monkeys that there are many cells in V1 that respond more to some wavelengths of light than others. This fact is simply missed by the BOLD response, because these different cells are close together and have the same requirements for oxygen. We cannot, therefore, with present evidence, exclude the possibility that cells in V1 contribute to the sensation of colour.

Perhaps they make a contribution, but only an unconscious one? Only when the signals reach the specialised colour area might the activity become conscious. This takes us into the tricky area of 'unconscious perception', the subject of the next (short) chapter.

14

Unconscious Perception

'Unconscious perception' sounds like a contradiction in terms, like 'military music', or 'scientific humour'; but psychologists have a robust definition, following the lead of Sigmund Freud: 'If you react to some stimulus but deny having seen it, it's unconscious.' For example, words are flashed briefly on to a TV screen and the observer's task is to press one button if the word is man-made (like 'hammer') and another if it is not ('river'). If 'hammer' is repeated twice in succession, the time to make the correct decision is smaller on the second occasion. This is true even if the second word is 'HAMMER' or *__hammer__*, so it is the similarity in the words' meaning rather than visual similarity that counts. This 'repetition priming' effect – as it is called – may seem obvious, but it works even if the first word is presented too quickly to be clearly perceived. (To ensure this, it is followed by a burst of random letters on the TV screen.) The observer is unable to name the first word, but repetition priming still works. According to psychologists, this means that the word was 'unconsciously perceived', or, if you want to be really pedantic, 'unconsciously processed up to the semantic level'.

Unconscious perception is the same as 'subliminal perception' – so called because it is below the threshold, or 'limen', for sensation. The wife of a US Presidential candidate believed that certain gramophone records contained subliminal satanic messages. Subliminal TV advertising was actually used by the Republican Party in the 2001 Presidential Election, where it seems to have been a failure, because the messages were consciously perceived. But how do we know whether 'subliminal' messages are consciously perceived or not? The obvious problem with 'unconscious' perception is that we have to take the observer's word for it (literally) that they did not consciously see the stimulus. Or do we? We could by-pass language by asking the observer to press one button if they perceived the stimulus, and another if they did not – it sounds straightforward, but a phenomenon dubbed 'blindsight' has thrown a large spanner in the works. The story of blindsight begins, once again, with brain-damaged patients.

Patients with complete damage of the primary visual cortex (V1) are blind, in the ordinary and legal sense of the term. They are unable to use their eyes to read, recognise colours or avoid obstacles. All this is predictable from anatomy, since the vast majority of the nerve fibres from the retina go to V1 before they go anywhere else. However, not all the nerve fibres from the optic nerve are routed through V1. Another pathway goes directly through the mid-brain (where the frog has its main visual brain, the optic tectum) and then goes back to the cerebral cortex. Can this meandering path be used for vision?

The British Army doctor G. Riddoch treated soldiers with head injuries during the First World War. Like Inouye before him, he found that localised injury to the primary visual cortex produced regions of localised blindness, or 'scotomata'. However, in some cases Riddoch noted that his patients could still see motion in their apparently blind field. His observations remained as a curiosity until further experiments on the 'residual vision' of men and monkeys in the 1970s. 'Residual vision' refers to the sparing of some functions inside a cortically blind area. For example, patients were able to move their eyes towards a light flash in their supposedly blind field. Later studies showed that they could press a button to indicate whether an object in the blind field was moving upwards or downwards.

There seems to be a paradox here. To understand what is going on, we have to look carefully at how the 'blindness' was measured in the first place. The devil is in the detail. Here is Inouye's description:

I moved the white test object of 10 mm² size in the Foerster perimeter and found several ring-shaped scotomata whose position changed between measurements. During the measurement, I asked the patient to say 'yes' if he noticed the white object and I would continue doing this, for example, 60⁰. 'Yes, yes, yes', and so forth until he said 'no'. Then at 56⁰ he said 'no, no, no', and so forth until again he said 'yes', etc., etc.

Like an eyewitness in a court of law, the patient is being asked to report what they themselves have seen: they are not to make any inferences about what they think may have really happened, or to make suppositions about what anyone else might have seen. It is their own subjective experience that is at issue, nothing more or less. The tests that reveal residual vision are very different. The patient is not asked whether or not they 'saw' something. Instead, a simple reaction is measured, such as an eye movement; or the patient is asked to 'guess' whether the stimulus is moving leftwards or rightwards. The important thing is that the patient is not allowed to say, 'Don't know – I can't see the stimulus.' They have to make a decision, a procedure technically known as 'forced choice'. So the problem in a nutshell is that the patient denies 'seeing' the stimulus in a 'yes–no' test, but can detect it in a forced-choice test, or by an eye movement.

Many thousands of words have been written on this topic, some of them quite acrimonious. The obvious problem is that we have no way of measuring awareness directly. Asking people is the most direct approach, but it assumes that people are always quite sure whether they are experiencing something or not. This is not true. In 'The Passing of Arthur', Tennyson describes with great precision these far margins of visual consciousness:

> Thereat once more he moved about, and clamb
> Ev'n to the highest he could climb and saw
> Straining his eye beneath an arch of hand
> Or thought he saw, the speck that bare the King,
> Down that long water opening on the deep
> Somewhere far off, pass on and on and go
> From less to less and vanish into light.
> And the new sun rose bringing the New Year.

The sensation of the speck that bore the King was uncertain, as is typical of weak or 'noisy' sensation. The presence of random activity in the nervous system makes it inevitable that observers will sometimes be unsure whether they have really seen something in the outside world, or not. When they say 'no' they mean that the evidence did not justify saying 'yes'; but it is still possible for this 'invisible' signal to have some other effect upon the observer, such as making the pupil of the eye contract, or betting that the stimulus is more likely to have moved up than down. This has suggested to psychologists a strategy for finding out which brain processes are conscious and which are not. If an unconsciously perceived message ('No') activates brain areas A and B, while a consciously perceived message ('Yes') activates areas A, B and C, then C is responsible for consciousness.

In an fMRI experiment using this logic, observers were tested in the repetition-priming experiment described earlier. 'Unconsciously perceived' words increased the activity in several brain areas, including those normally involved in reading, but 'consciously perceived' words also activated an area called the 'prefrontal cortex', one of the candidate areas (as we shall see later) for the seat of consciousness. However, the 'conscious' words also caused greater activity in the 'reading areas' than did the unconscious words. Perhaps the reading areas have to reach a sufficient level of activity before the observer will report seeing the word ('Yes'). Another problem is that the observers were never asked how confident they were that the words were 'unconscious'. Given the chance, they might have said something like 'I'm not at all certain, but I think there may have been a very quick flash.' Perhaps the distinction between conscious and unconscious is a red herring, and it is all a matter of degree – like the strength of the BOLD response. Tennyson may have been a better psychologist than the latter-day followers of Sigmund Freud after all.

So far, then, we have failed to find special areas of the brain that 'light up' only when we are conscious. What would it mean, in any case, to say that some parts of the brain are conscious, and others not? Is there some special property of conscious nerve cells, that makes them identifiable under a microscope, like liver cells? The next chapter looks further at the strange idea that conscious nerve cells 'secrete' sensations.

15

The Secretion Theory of Consciousness

'When Cabanis said that thought was a function of the brain, in the same sense as bile secretion is a function of the liver, he blundered philosophically,' wrote Thomas Henry Huxley to the Reverend E. McGlure in 1891. Huxley was referring to the French philosopher and physiologist Pierre Jean George Cabanis (1757–1808). Spotting the nature of Cabanis's alleged blunder is not rocket science. Bile is produced by a particular kind of cell in the body. We can trace the biochemical pathways that make bile-producing cells different from other cells. Special genes are activated in these cells to make the manufacture of bile possible; yet as far as we know, there is no biochemical pathway for the manufacture of a 'red' sensation. The analogy between bile and sensation breaks down.

It is true that the brain contains hundreds, if not thousands, of different cell types, varying in shape from the 'starburst amacrine cell' of the retina to the 'mossy fibres' in the cerebellum. Equally diverse are the biochemical mechanisms that cells use to communicate with one another: the neurotransmitters glutamate, acetylcholine, serotonin, GABA, ATP, nitric oxide – the roll-call lengthens inexorably with every meeting of the Society for Neuroscience. The diversity of cell types and biochemistry presumably explains why many human genes are expressed only in the brain. Yet there is no evidence that different cell types secrete different sensations. The grey matter of all mammals has the same basic six-layered structure all over the brain, and contains the same cell types. A microscope gives us no answer to the question why one area is 'visual' and another 'auditory'; nor does the crackling electrical output of nerve cells amplified by a loudspeaker tell us whether the cells are seeing or hearing.

To be sure, there are small differences in microscopic structures

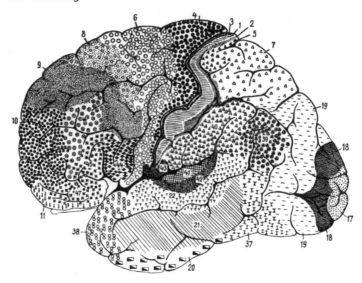

Figure 15.1 Brodmann's map of the human brain

across the grey matter of the cerebral hemispheres, used by the anatomist Brodmann in 1908 to divide grey matter into roughly fifty different areas, such as the 'striate cortex' area 17 (see figure 15.1); but area 17 looks different from other areas mainly because of the huge swathe of fat-covered nerve fibres entering it from the optic tract, rather than because it contains a particular kind of cell. A tenable hypothesis about grey matter holds that it is basically the same everywhere and contains the same basic cell types, connected in the same way.

It is a fairly safe bet, then, that the secretion theory is wrong. Even if we could find a particular cell or group of cells that fired when, and only when, we had a sensation of 'red', it is not the structure of these cells themselves that explains the sensation. As one colour scientist put it: 'Colours are so gay that those with total colour loss cannot but be pitied; and it must be wondered what it is that makes red produce the wonderful red sensation most people perceive.' There is an obvious and well-trodden alternative to the secretion theory. Any cells that fire specifically to 'red' surfaces are just a small part of the ebb and flow of information from the surface of outside objects to the actions of the organism. A monkey foraging for a red fruit amongst green leaves is not interested in the wavelength of light, but in finding the right fruit to eat. The wavelength of light reflected from the fruit changes when the sun goes behind a cloud, but the surface of the fruit itself does not change. Therefore, true colour perception must take account of the state of the lighting – a complicated and difficult computation. To classify a part of the image as 'green' is to assign it to the heteroclitic category of objects that are green – for example, leaves. 'Red', 'blue' and 'green' are not simple secretions of nerve cells, but complex concepts involving memory, emotion and readiness for action. This may be why neuroscientists have failed so far to discover nerve cells 'tuned' to the pure colours such as red and green. Colours must have meaning, or colour vision would not have evolved. The earliest fish to distinguish the shorter wavelengths of light from the rest of the spectrum did so because 'blue' light comes from above, and their genes are in our blood. Blue is considered a more distant colour than red – a fact unexplained by the idea that it is a simple secretion.

In other words, we see colour when our brain classifies part of the retinal image as coming from a surface of a particular type. This act of classification is impossible without a key set of cells in a small area (perhaps V4), but that does not mean that these cells secrete special sensations. 'Colour cells' owe their powers of discrimination to their connections with other cells, earlier in the visual pathway. 'Green' cells are no greener than 'red' cells and probably have identical anatomy and chemistry. However, this does not mean that it is foolish to look for parts of the brain that have the function of classifying colours. (Similarly, we can ask which member of the rugby team is the blind-side wing forward, without supposing that there is anything in his physical appearance that gives him that function.) Indeed, it is often a very practical question, particularly when people experience sensations that 'leak' from one sense to another. For example, some blind patients see flashes of light in the 'blind' area when they are startled by sounds varying from walls 'crackling' at night to a pencil striking the desk. Sensations varied from 'simple flashes of white light' to complicated colourful hallucinations likened to a flame, a petal of oscillating lines, a kaleidoscope or an amoeba; they always appeared within a defective portion of the visual field as demonstrated by perimetry. It is perfectly reasonable to ask where in the patient's brain these visual sensations happen.

Clearly, it is no longer in the retina alone, since this has been disconnected from the brain in the blind area. We can consider two different kinds of explanation. One is that nerve cells in the part of the brain stimulated by sounds have suddenly become capable of producing visual sensations. This is hard to credit. What possible changes in their structure could have produced such a change? How could the same cells produce both visual and auditory sensations? A better bet is that the nerve impulses in the 'sound pathway' are somehow leaking into the normal visual pathway, and are causing sensations of light in the visual nerve cells where such sensations normally occur.

A possible site for leakage of sounds into the visual pathway is the small many-layered structure known to anatomists as the 'lateral geniculate nucleus'. (It gets its name from its knee-like appearance). Nerve fibres from the retina terminate their journey here, and the messages running along them are transferred to a further pathway – the optic tract – that takes them up to the primary visual cortex. The geniculate is a much-studied but little-understood structure. It used to be thought of as a mere 'relay station', though the implied analogy with a telegraph is not a good one, since nerve impulses do not diminish in strength with distance. We now know that most of the nerve fibres entering the lateral geniculate come not from the optic tract at all, but from the grey matter to which it supposedly 'projects'. Some of these 'down-flowing' fibres may be activated by sound. Normally, their signals may be too weak to be effective; but if the cells there are deprived of their normal visual input they may become more sensitive to other inputs. Such an effect has been observed in nerve cells of the spinal cord. There is direct evidence that sounds produce activity in nerve cells of the LGN, even in normal monkeys.

Sounds can produce visual sensation even in normal observers. In the right circumstances, a sound presented at the same time as a single light flash causes that flash to be seen as *two* flashes, not one. The stage is now set for finding out exactly where in the brain this 'doubled' visual sensation first starts, using rapid brain-imaging techniques. If we found the 'doubled response' in the lateral geniculate and the primary visual cortex we should not have learned much. However, it would be much more interesting if we found the doubled response only in the temporal lobe. We would then suspect that nerve impulses do not cause sensations until they progress beyond the primary visual cortex. The idea of this research is to drive sensations into a smaller and smaller space in the brain, like rabbits cornered by a combine harvester.

Some philosophers and psychologists deplore the search for sensations in the brain and think it silly. Their favourite dismissive phrase is 'the category error', a term introduced by philosopher Gilbert Ryle in his influential book *The Concept of Mind*. Ryle was a brilliant polemicist who coined the term 'ghost in the machine' to lampoon the idea that the brain contains some special mind-substance. His book accomplishes the amazing feat of discussing the concept of mind without the benefit of a single scientific fact. According to Ryle, a category error is being committed by someone who sees a body of marching soldiers and says, 'Yes, a fine body of men, but where is the regiment?'; and according to Ryle's followers, it is a category error to ask, 'Where is the sensation of red located?' However, this objection to localisation of function is puzzling. The regiment may be no different from the men comprising it, but it has a localisation in space, and it makes perfect sense for a lost soldier to say, 'I am looking for the Gloucestershires.' If we believe that sensations and brain events are *one and the same thing*, we are not making a category error, but avoiding one. In any case, the logic of the double sensation makes perfect sense as an experimental programme in neuroscience, whatever problems it might cause for our inadequate language faculty.

Like collectors of rare stamps, neuroscientists looking for conscious brain mechanisms hope that they will be few in number. Francis Crick and Christoff Koch take the bold step of eliminating the whole of the primary visual cortex (V1) from their enquiries. V1, they say, is an entirely *unconscious* mechanism; visual sensations take place elsewhere, and 'elsewhere' is the prefrontal cortex at the front of the brain. This idea is especially appealing to those who think that there is some fundamental difference between man and monkey. The primary visual cortex of the macaque monkey, the most studied species, shows no obviously important difference in organisation from that of man; but the prefrontal cortex of man has enormously expanded. As a consequence, the visual areas of the macaque take up almost half of its cerebral cortex, while in man they amount to only about 30 per cent.

The first point Crick and Koch make is that normal observers cannot tell whether a flash of light in a dark room is presented to the left or the right eye. We can, however, tell whether we are being touched on the left or the right hand. Why the difference? A convincing explanation is that (as far as we know) all the cells in grey matter *except V1* have equal connections to the two eyes. Looking at the firing of these cells, we cannot tell which eye is being stimulated. Cells responding to touch, however, are different for the left and right hands. (Indeed, they are on opposite sides of the brain.) The logical follow-up to this argument is that sensation does not take place in V1 itself, since millions of cells there *are* able to distinguish between the left and right eye.

Because left and right eye cells give rise to apparently indistinguishable sensations, Crick and Koch argue that the striate cortex does not contribute 'directly' to conscious experience. However, it is a little difficult to know here what they mean by 'directly'. They seem to be saying that left and right eye cells do not secrete different sensations, but this is to attack a straw man. The secretion theorist is not obliged to say that different cells always secrete a different sensation, only that different sensations are always secreted by different cells. (T. H. Huxley understood this point perfectly when he said that sensation is a *function* of the brain, in the mathematical sense.) If a cell in the left eye and a cell in the right eye point towards the same position in space and detect the same changes there, why should they produce different secretions? We simply have to say that left- and right-eye cells have identical functions and can substitute for one another in the causal chain leading to perception.

In other words, if we found a normal observer who could tell which eye was being stimulated, we would have to invent a pathway in which the two eyes were kept separate. A male observer AJ may have had such a pathway. He wore no correcting lenses, and had no optical differences between the eyes, such as astigmatism. He had normal stereoscopic acuity, and no defect in colour vision in either eye was revealed by the Ishihara plates; but he could discriminate perfectly between his two eyes. He was quite unable to give an account of his unusual skill, saying that it was just 'obvious' to him which eye was being stimulated. Either he was using some very subtle cue, such as difference of focus between the two eyes, or he was using some previously unknown anatomical pathway or mechanism leading from one-eyed cells to higher levels and preserving the difference between them.

The rabbit, with its eyes on the side of its head, presumably finds it easy to know which eye is being stimulated when a fox is approaching from the left-hand side. The images in the rabbit's two eyes are like a panoramic photograph, the parts of which are 'stitched' in its brain. If two very different images are presented to the human eyes, our experience is entirely different from that of the rabbit, because our eyes point forward rather than sideways. Instead of a panorama, we experience conflict between the two images – a condition called 'binocular rivalry', currently one of the very hot areas of research in visual neuroscience. When rivalry is occurring, we tend to see only one eye's image at a time. After a while, this conscious image fades out and we see the image in the other eye, and so on. Each eye's view lasts for several seconds. If we could find cells in the brain that increased and decreased their activity in exact synchrony with our perceptions, we would be justified – the argument runs – in saying that they make a 'direct' contribution to consciousness. Conversely, the argument continues, if other cells show no relation to the changes in perceptions, we could exclude them from the conscious process.

Rivalry is illustrated by the images composed of coloured rings illustrated in the plate section. The two images can be superimposed by crossing the eyes ('squinting'). Once the rings are fused, several facts about rivalry become clear. First, the colours seen in the display are unstable. Parts of the outer ring, in particular, are sometimes seen as red and sometimes, a few seconds later, as green. Second, the parts of the outer ring do not always change colour at the same time. One sector may be seen as red while another sector is seen as green. Thus, rivalry between the eyes is not settled by switching one eye entirely off, but by competition within patches, like the map after a parliamentary election. Third, the outer and inner ring are seen at different distances (depths) because they are at slightly different relative positions in the two eyes. This is the phenomenon of binocular stereopsis. For depth perception, the competition between the eyes is settled not by rivalry, but by mutual co-operation. This is lucky, or we should be experiencing rivalry all the time from the slight geometrical differences of the image between the eyes. Co-operation for computing depth co-exists with competition between colours. This is a beautifully simple demonstration that the different qualities of the retinal image – in this case its colour and its shape – are computed by different mechanisms in the brain. Finally, some observers may see a degree of colour-mixing between the eyes: the small inner ring is seen neither as red nor as green, but as a muddy reddish-yellow.

Rivalry can also be seen in the textures illustrated in figure 15.2. If the images on the top are flashed very quickly, one to the left eye and one to the right, observers can see that there is a square in the bottom-left-hand corner, despite the fact that the tilts of the lines in the two eyes go in opposite directions. Observers report a paradoxical perception: they can see the square, but they see no difference between the lines inside and outside its boundary – in other words, they see a boundary between two textures that are the same! The brain, like a true artist, can entertain contradictory notions without going mad.

Left Eye   Right Eye

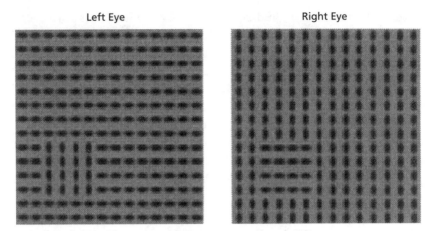

Figure 15.2 The 'pop-out' square (left) can still be identified when the two eyes' images are perceptually fused

This demonstration implies that the square is seen in V1, where the inputs from the two eyes are still partly separate.

Rivalry may seem to argue that V1 does, after all, make a 'direct contribution' to awareness. How could we cut out one eye's image from our consciousness unless we first suppressed it in the 'monocular' cells of V1? Unfortunately, things are not so simple. After all, if we put on a piratical eyepatch we see through one eye only, but this does not mean that perception happens in that eye. Rivalry might be no more than the equivalent of an eyepatch in V1. If this is so, the choice between rivalrous perceptions might be taking place not in V1 at all, but in 'higher' levels of the visual brain. A demonstration supporting this was discovered by the Spanish oculist Diaz-Caneja of Palencia in 1928 (see plate section). The left-hand side of the left-eye image and the right-hand side of the right-eye image can be combined to give a complete image of parallel lines. Likewise, the curved lines can be combined to produce circles. Diaz-Caneja found that his observers experienced rivalry between lines and circles, not between left and right eyes. In other words, rivalry is not between eyes at all, but between different perceptual interpretations, as in ambiguous figures such as the duck-rabbit. Unfortunately, not even this argument is conclusive. We already know from the coloured-rings image (plate section) that rivalry is patchy, and this may be what is happening in the Diaz-Caneja figure. In fact, observers report all sorts of combinations of left and right half in addition to pure lines or pure circles, such as spirals from a combination of straight lines, circles, and junctions between lines and circles. The evidence of Diaz-Caneja's figure is interesting, but not quite conclusive.

These arguments are complicated, and it is tempting once again to cut the Gordian knot with brain imaging. Surely it would be easy to find out whether left-eye cells in the visual cortex are silenced when the right eye dominates? The history starts strangely enough, with experiments on the nervous system of plants by Charles Darwin at his home in Down House. Darwin spent a considerable part of his time staring at plants in his garden, leading his gardener to proclaim that his master's notoriously weak health would be improved if he found himself some useful work to occupy his mind. Darwin was especially fascinated by the response of the Venus flytrap to touch. The snapping shut of the plant around its insect prey seemed similar to that of an animal with a nervous system: perhaps animals and plants were descendants of a common ancestor with a primitive nervous system; but where were the nerve cells of the plant? Lacking the necessary apparatus to test his idea, Darwin handed the problem over to John Burdon-Sanderson, a professor of physiology at University College, London and an ancestor of the irascible geneticist J. B. S. Haldane. Burdon-Sanderson was able to measure small electrical potentials in the plant travelling at the very slow speed of 3 cm/sec. (We now know that these are carried not along nerves, but by current passing directly through small holes called 'plasmodesmata' in the cell walls of the plant.) The problem of plant sensation was later taken up by the Indian physicist and physiologist Sir Jagadis Chunder Bose (1858–1937), who studied the electro-optical response of plants to light stimulation. Bose later applied his techniques to the human retina, where he discovered what we now call the 'electro-optogram', or wave of electrical activity following light stimulation. He also observed that after-images provoked by a flash of intense light lasted for tens of seconds, but seemed to fade in and out of consciousness. While this was going on, the electroretinogram seemed to be out of step in the two eyes. Was the explanation of binocular rivalry to be found in the eye itself?

Bose's idea that rivalry starts in the eye has had no support from later research. The results of electrical recording from the brain contradict one another with the regularity of binocular rivalry itself. In 1964 an experiment used electrodes on the scalp to measure the response of the human visual cortex to a flickering light in one eye.

The brain wave followed the flicker at 8 waves per second. When a striped pattern was placed in the other eye there were periods when it dominated the flickering pattern, and during these periods the brain wave following the flicker was reduced by over 80 per cent. The experiment seemed to prove conclusively that suppression was happening in the visual cortex – presumably by competition between 'left-eye' and 'right-eye' neurones. A problem with scalp recording is that it is not very good at localising the signal in the brain. Recording from single nerve cells in animals can give more precise coordinates. Here again, an experiment in 1964 in cats found that the response of cells to bars in one eye was suppressed by suddenly presenting bars tilted at 90 degrees in the other eye. Functional MRI scans can also pinpoint V1 accurately enough to tell us whether rivalry is occurring there. A recent experiment exploited the fact that the BOLD response is roughly proportional to the contrast of the visual stimulus. Observers viewed a low-contrast pattern of vertical stripes in one eye and a higher-contrast pattern of horizontal stripes in the other eye. Because of the difference in the angle of the stripes between the eyes, the observers experienced binocular rivalry; and when they did so, the BOLD response in V1 was higher during the periods when they were experiencing the high-contrast pattern.

Despite this apparently conclusive evidence for rivalry in V1, other experiments disagree. In one such, monkeys were first trained to press on a lever for a reward when tilted bars changed their tilt by 90 degrees in the same eye. They were then shown bars 90 degrees out of register in the two eyes – a stimulus that evokes conscious rivalry in the human observer between the two directions of tilt. The stimulus on the retinas was unchanging, but the monkey continued to press the lever from time to time as if it were seeing a change in tilt. The next step was to record from individual cells in the monkey's brain while it was reporting its perceptions. If suppression is happening in cells of the primary visual cortex, we would expect their firing to wax and wane in step with the changes in perception. The experiment gave no clear evidence for this. Other cells, downstream in the visual pathway, did wax and wane in the expected way, but there was no evident pattern to the results. Some cells preferred 45-degree stripes and responded more when the monkey was reported seeing 45-degree stripes than when it was seeing 135-degree stripes. This is as expected, but other cells showed exactly the reverse pattern, responding more when the monkey was not reporting their preferred tilt.

Sauce for the goose is sauce for the gander. Other experiments, on cells in the prefrontal cortex, have shown no correlation between their activity and the monkey's perceptions. If V1 is an unconscious automaton, the same logic should lead us to exclude the prefrontal cortex from awareness. All in all, if the primary visual cortex stood accused in a Scottish court of law of being an unconscious automaton, a jury would almost certainly return the verdict 'not proven' from the evidence given so far. Rivalry is not sufficiently conclusive. Even if we were persuaded that nerve cells in V1 show no changes during rivalry related to change in conscious state, we could not conclude that they were unconscious. The states of mind alternating in rivalry have just as much in common as they have in competition. The idea that V1 neurones make no 'direct' contribution to awareness makes sense only in the context of the secretion theory, which we can reject anyway on logical grounds.

The secretion theory of consciousness says that our conscious experiences are associated with the activity of a privileged set of nerve cells in the brain. Retinal cells make no contribution to awareness, according to this theory. Nor, according to Crick and Koch, does activity in the primary visual cortex make a 'direct' contribution to experience. The logical problem here is that nothing in the physical structure of nerve cells gives any clue as to why only some of them but not others should secrete consciousness. The alternative to the secretion theory is that consciousness is explained by the flow of information through nerve cells from the outside world to our actions and decisions. If this view is correct, we cannot take the brain to pieces like a car engine and say, 'Consciousness occurs *here* in these particular nerve cells.' Despite this, many neuroscientists remain wedded to the idea that we can dissect consciousness out of the brain. Their argument runs that it may be difficult to understand why some cells but not others contribute to awareness, but at least we can classify cells into conscious and unconscious varieties. The final chapter will describe further attacks on V1, and a remarkable theory that many of our actions – such as reaching for an object – are under the control of an unconscious machine.

16

Into the Mill

The philosopher Gottfried Wilhelm von Leibniz (1646–1716) rebutted localisation of consciousness in his metaphor of the mill:

> If we imagine that there is a machine whose structure makes it think, sense, and have perceptions, we could conceive it enlarged, having the same proportions, so that we could enter it, as one enters into a mill. Assuming that, when inspecting its interior, we will only find parts that push against each other, and we will never find anything to explain the perception. (G. W. Leibniz, *The Monadology*)

The problem with Leibniz's argument is that it assumes the truth of its conclusion in its premise – the error called *petitio principi* in the medieval schools. First we are told to imagine a machine whose structure makes it have sensations, and then we are told that such a machine is impossible! Leibniz is saying that, when we enter the giant mill of another's brain, what we perceive there will be our own perceptions, not those of the brain we have entered. When a person is perceiving the colour red, we do not expect red-perceiving cells in their brain to glow in that colour. To that extent Leibniz is clearly right; but what we find in the mill may well *explain* the perceptions of that brain completely. That, at least, is the premise of most neuroscientists, who hope to find that some parts of the mill are more important than others in explaining what it perceives. They call this (rather pompously) the search for 'neural correlates of consciousness'. Latter-day followers of Leibniz, on the other hand, continue to say that a machine for producing consciousness cannot be divided into 'conscious' and 'unconscious' parts.

The map in the primary visual cortex (V1) has become the battlefield for this new philosophical conflict. We know for certain that the map in V1 is accurate enough to pinpoint the direction of objects in space; it contains cells tuned to the third dimension (distance), and cells with preferences for size and the tilt of objects; but is V1 conscious – or does it merely contribute information to 'higher levels', where consciousness truly occurs? The accusation that V1 is an unconscious automaton gets some support, but not much, from binocular rivalry (see previous chapter). However, there is further evidence against the accused. One line of enquiry is the waterfall illusion – seen after we stare at a moving texture for a few minutes. Stationary texture then seems to move in the opposite direction to the so-called 'adapting stimulus'. We now combine the waterfall effect with binocular rivalry. If we adapt to a downwards-moving texture in the left eye at the same time as an upwards-moving texture in the right eye, we experience 'binocular rivalry' – sometimes we see the upwards movement and sometimes the downwards. If we then look at stationary texture through the left eye, it seems to move upwards – the opposite of the direction it saw previously; and similarly for the right eye. We conclude that separate and opposite adaptation can occur in the two eyes, and that adaptation therefore occurs in V1 – the only area both sensitive to movement direction and containing 'monocular cells' connected to one eye only. But here is the crunch: adaptation of the left eye during rivalry does not depend on the length of time the observer *experiences* the downwards movement – it depends only on the time it was present on the retina. It seems that adaptation of left-eye nerve cells in V1 is happening even during times when we are unaware of the stimulus in that eye. The adapting cells there cannot be the 'neural correlates of consciousness' after all, and adaptation is a purely unconscious process.

Another example comes from the phenomenon of 'crowding' illustrated in figure 16.1. If we look at a single letter 'K' in the periphery of our vision we can easily read it, but if it is surrounded by other letters, it becomes illegible. This so-called 'crowding' effect has given rise to controversy about the fairness of the driving test. Drivers are supposed to be able to read a car number plate from 25 yards. When this test was devised, number plates had only six letters – for example, AJA 985 (the number of my old family car, a Standard 8). Now they have one more letter, crammed into the same space. This makes them harder to read at 25 yards, particularly for observers with certain clinical conditions, such as amblyopia. It is only a matter of time before someone challenges their exclusion from driving by the 25-yard test with the modern number plate.

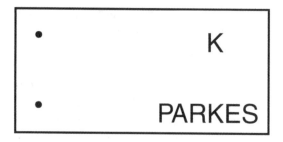

Figure 16.1 A demonstration of 'crowding'

If crowding is severe, observers cannot tell whether a target line is tilted horizontally (–) or vertically (I), when it is surrounded by other tilted lines. This is where the neural correlates of consciousness in V1 can be put to the test. We know that many single cells in V1 have preferences for the tilt of lines: if they are the neural correlates of our perception of tilt, we expect their preferences to be wiped out by crowding. To test this prediction, observers were instructed to stare for several minutes at an image containing a tilted line surrounded by crowding lines. Because of the crowding they were unable to say whether the target line was horizontal or vertical. After this period of adaptation, the observer's sensitivity for detecting lines was measured in the part of the image previously occupied by the target line. The usual result of adapting to a tilted line is that it becomes harder to detect a line of the same tilt as the target. Adaptation is normally explained by some form of fatigue in nerve cells repeatedly exposed to the same stimulus; but what if the line were invisible at the time of adaptation? It makes little difference, the experimenters found. After adaptation to a vertical line, observers were less sensitive to vertical lines, even though they were unable to say whether the adapting stimulus itself was horizontal or vertical. The explanation? Adaptation takes place in V1, like the waterfall effect, but adaptation is an unconscious process. The 'tilted cells' in V1 provide the information allowing higher areas to compute the tilt of lines, but are themselves unconscious of tilt, like secret agents who pass on coded messages, which to them have no meaning.

Clearly, then, the firing of cells in V1 is not *sufficient* for our conscious visual awareness; but have we really learned anything new from these experiments? A Leibnizian sceptic might say not, and that we have merely succeeded, yet again., in refuting a straw man – the secretion theory. Of course, activity of a single cell in V1 could not secrete a conscious experience of line tilt! The cells 'tuned' to vertical have the same shape and biochemistry as those tuned to horizontal, so it would be totally mysterious if they were to produce different sensations. Moreover, we know that cells 'tuned' to vertical respond almost as vigorously to lines slightly tilted away from vertical, but we do not experience mixtures of tilt sensations when we see a vertical line. As a matter of logic, it must be the pattern of activity over *many cells* that causes perception of tilt. We do not get round this problem by imagining a single cell at a higher level that responds *only* to vertical lines. Unless this cell has a different shape or biochemistry from other cells, it would be irrational to suppose that it secretes consciousness all by itself. It must in turn be its connections, both upstream and downstream, that give its firing a meaning. The analogy with secret agents and coded messages is misleading, because it presupposes the existence of a conscious 'M' sitting in the brain decoding messages from her agents – in other words, a 'ghost in the machine'.

So the evidence to convict V1 of insentience is still inconclusive. What about blindsight – the condition in which patients with damage to V1 can react to stimuli, but apparently have no conscious awareness of them? Does blindsight prove that V1 is *necessary* for awareness, as some have claimed? Unfortunately, this argument hinges on the proposition that blindsight patients are truly unaware, and this is difficult (if not impossible) to prove. Opponents of blindsight say that the residual vision of patients is a conscious process. One especially well-studied blindsight patient, GY, has given contradictory results in different laboratories, albeit with slightly different stimuli. A recent psychophysical study of GY asked him to say how certain he was that he had seen, or not seen, the stimulus on each trial, using a four-point 'confidence scale'. A normal observer is more likely to make a correct 'yes' response on trials when they are 'sure' than on trials when they are 'unsure'. This was true of GY as well, indicating that he knew what he was up to. On the other hand, the correlation was not as strong as it is in normal observers, suggesting that GY has difficulty in labelling the strength of his sensations.

Another line of attack on the problem of GY's awareness has been to see if he can match the appearance of images in his 'blind' field of vision to other images in his normal field. If he can do so, the argument runs, he must be having conscious experience of these stimuli. A 'thought experiment' may help to make the logic of this procedure clear. Suppose we have a red–green colour-blind observer whose defect is confined to one eye. We want to know whether he is capable of having sensations of red through his colour-blind eye. The experiment is to have him look at a patch of colour in the normal eye that he calls 'red'. We now present a second patch of colour in the colour-blind eye and allow the observer to adjust its wavelength until it looks exactly the same as the colour in the normal eye. If the observer can do this, we infer that he can have 'normal sensations of red in the colour-blind eye.

The equivalent for blindsight is to show the observer some image in their 'blind' field, and to see if there is stimulus in their normal field that evokes the same sensation. For example, would the observer accept a match between a rapidly moving, high-contrast bar in the blind field and a slowly moving, low-contrast bar? In many cases the answer was no; but not in all cases: for example, moving textures of low contrast were accepted to match moving bars in the other eye. We may conclude that GY has at least some sensations in his 'blind field', although the experiment does not conclusively prove that the experience was visual. GY could have matched the stimuli on the basis of some non-visual sensation arising from stimuli in both the normal and blind fields. It is not unknown for stimuli in one sense modality to evoke sensations in another, as we have seen in the case of auditory-visual synaesthesia. Blind people using echo-sounders to move about sometimes say that they experience the feedback as light touches to the face, rather than as sounds.

So far, then, we seem to have failed to run down visual awareness to any particular part of the visual pathway. V1 has been under sustained attack, accused of being an unconscious automaton, but has narrowly survived. What about other divisions of the brain? A very bold attempt to dissect consciousness out of the visual brain has recently been based on the distinction between pathways responsible for 'visual action' and pathways responsible for 'seeing'. The distinction has its origin in Ferrier's mistaken identification of the angular gyrus of the parietal lobe as the seat of visual sensation. Ferrier thought that his monkeys were blind after removal of the angular gyrus, but it later became clear that it was their ability to reach and pick up objects that was impaired, not their visual sensitivity as such. In 1982 Glickstein and May reviewed this and other literature and came to the conclusion that there are two very different streams of visual processing issuing from the striate cortex (V1). A 'dorsal stream' leads upwards from V1 towards the parietal lobe, and ultimately to the pons and cerebellum, where it is involved in the control of action. A 'ventral stream' leads downwards to the temporal lobe, where objects are recognised and categorised (see plate section). At the same time Mishkin and Ungerleider independently developed the idea that there are two streams: a ventral stream for object recognition and a dorsal stream for space: the 'what?' and 'where?' pathways.

A recent idea, from two neuropsychologists, Milner and Goodale, is that visual awareness is associated with the ventral pathway alone. The dorsal pathway is an unconscious automaton, useful for running down a flight of stairs, but not involved in conscious vision. The evidence comes from a patient DF, who has 'visual form agnosia' – the condition similar to the one dramatised by Oliver Sachs in his book *The Man who mistook his Wife for a Hat*. DF has more or less intact ability to detect when objects appear in her visual field and has a strong sense of colour. She is, in this respect, totally different from patients with 'cortical blindness' arising from damage to V1. But she is very poor indeed at recognising shapes, even ones as simple as squares and rectangles. She is reasonably good with natural objects such as fruit and vegetables, possibly because she can use colour and texture, rather than outline shape. Her deficit is most apparent with line drawings of objects, which she can neither name nor copy (see figure 16.2).

The precise nature of DF's brain damage is unknown because it

Figure 16.2 Fig. 5.2 Drawings by patient DF

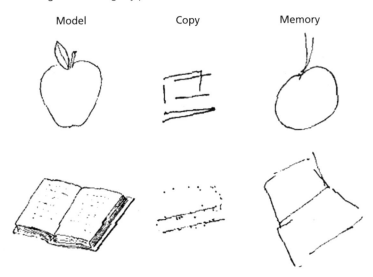

resulted from carbon monoxide poisoning, which causes widespread cell damage. A scan shortly after her accident suggested that the striate cortex was undamaged; but the same scan showed damage in the visual areas surrounding the striate cortex: V2, V3 and V4. However, the damage is not complete and it may be more accurate to think in terms of a loss of particular kinds of cell, rather than complete regions of the brain. Carbon monoxide damages cells by depriving them of oxygen, and some cells may be more tolerant of this than others. The loss of form perception recalls Inouye's patient Mr Tanaka, who could name a cup or a book correctly, but not most other things. However, Mr Tanaka lost his ability to name colours, which is not the case with DF.

Even more striking than DF's loss of form perception are her remaining abilities. 'DF . . . recovered within weeks,' the investigators report, 'the ability to reach out and grasp everyday objects.' She adjusts her grip appropriately to the object even before touching it, proving that she does have information about three-dimensional shape. In many ways, DF's disorder is the reverse of the one we met earlier in optic ataxia, where verbal object recognition is accurate, but the control of action is impaired. One experiment provides a peculiarly striking illustration of DF's condition. She was given a 'letter' to post through a slot that could be rotated around the clock face. This she did as accurately as a person without brain damage, rotating her hand and wrist to the correct angle before posting the letter. But if asked to *describe* the angle of the slot (horizontal, vertical or 45 degrees, for example) she was quite unable to do so. Actions speak louder than words for DF. Nor could she adjust the angle of a comparison slot to match that of the letter box. So it is not just her ability to name objects that is impaired, but rather her ability to *symbolise* objects abstractly, as opposed to reacting to them directly. These facts become more comprehensible if we say that DF has a problem with miming. Even for normal people, miming is an art that requires a great deal of practice to become perfect. Some actions are easier to mime than others – facial expressions, for example. Even young infants can mimic facial expressions, suggesting that the skill is 'hard-wired'. It would be interesting to see if DF preserves these skills.

Optic ataxia, the reverse of DF's condition, results from damage to areas of the parietal lobe in the dorsal 'action' pathway. Milner and Goodale make the suggestion that this action pathway is more or less intact in DF. Her real problem, they suggest, is in the ventral pathway leading to the temporal lobe, where the circuits for object recognition are thought to be located. Now comes the really surprising idea: that DF has no conscious experience of 'seeing'. Conscious experience, Milner and Goodale claim, resides in the ventral pathway. The dorsal action pathway is an unconscious automaton, devoted to action rather than experience. It is best to let the authors express this idea in their own words: 'Visual phenomenology, in our view, can arise only from processing in the ventral stream, processing that we have linked with recognition and perception. We have assumed in contrast that visual processing modules in the dorsal stream, despite the complex computations demanded by their role in the control of action, are not normally available to awareness.'

Who is telling us this? Not the action pathway, to be sure! The language centres are telling us that only abstract symbolic thought is truly conscious, not those dumb old motor pathways. Well, to paraphrase Mandy Rice-Davis, they would, wouldn't they? The huddled masses of the dorsal pathway need a champion to put their point of view into words. The first point to be made in their favour is that it requires a lot of special pleading to say that the agnosic has no conscious representation of objects. DF is quite well able to name natural objects, such as fruit and vegetables. It is all very well to say that she is doing this by looking at the texture, or by using other tricks; and it is also quite likely that texture is analysed without the help of the temporal lobe, perhaps even in the striate cortex itself, or in cells of one of the 'V' areas that has not been entirely destroyed by the carbon monoxide. But what becomes then of the claim that only the temporal lobe is conscious? It is stretching things more than a bit to say that the patient can name a Brussels sprout without having any awareness of what she has seen. Excuses could be multiplied but, as Aldous Huxley said, several excuses are always less convincing than one.

An even more compelling point is that DF is able to describe the positions of objects in space. She can *say* whether the red block is to the left or the right of the white block. The most reasonable inference from this ability, and from her unimpaired capacity to reach for and manipulate objects, is that her conscious representation of personal space is basically unimpaired. If she can do the left–right task, she can presumably also say whether the top of a tilted line is to the left or the right of its bottom. What she cannot do, apparently, is to look at two such tilted lines and say which of the two is tilted more in the clockwise direction. To understand this, we need to look more closely at the capacities of normal observers to do 'tilt discrimination' and what it involves. If the normal observer sees a tilted line, and several seconds later another tilted line, she can decide accurately which of them is more tilted (clockwise), provided they differ by about 1 degree. There must be some form of signal in the brain that outlasts the exposure of the first line, and which permits comparison of its tilt with that of the signal from the second line. Presumably these signals are in the form of nerve action potentials or states of cell membranes. The task of comparing the two noisy signals is not trivial, and presumably involves some specialised analogue machinery. Suppose the latter were damaged in the agnosic patient. They would have a perfectly intact visual awareness of both of the lines, but be unable to compare them. I am not saying that this is the true explanation of the deficit, only that it is a possible one. If it is correct, the problems of the object-agnosic may turn out to be a collection of highly specialised difficulties, rather than a panoptic loss of awareness.

Another problem with the automaton theory comes from a brain imaging study of 'neglect'. An invisible or 'extinguished' face in the neglected region of space continues to activate an area of the temporal lobe normally activated by visible faces. Thus activity in the face area of the temporal lobe is not *sufficient* for conscious experience. There is, as always with neuro-imaging, a caveat. The BOLD response gives only a very crude picture of what is happening in an area. The response of the face area to conscious and unconscious faces may not be the same, even if it appears the same in the BOLD response. Different nerve cells may be involved, or different patterns of nerve impulses.

There is one final objection to the theory that the dorsal stream is an automaton, and it comes from the monkey. When, over thirty years ago, recordings were made of 'object-recognition' nerve cells in the ventral pathway, the monkeys were anaesthetised. Unconsciousness seems to make no difference to the activity of these cells, so it is rather hard to argue that they are necessary and sufficient for awareness. The properties of cells in the dorsal pathway, on the other hand, have been established in awake, behaving monkeys.

Conclusion

The Search for the Grail

It seems that the search for the Holy Grail of neuroscience is in some disarray, with the Knights of the Round Table rushing about in different directions, claiming to have found the Grail in the most unlikely places. Some are no doubt tilting at windmills, to mix metaphors. Will we know when they have reached the end of their quest? Searching for consciousness is not quite the same as looking for a new atomic particle, the mass, spin and charge of which are predicted. A large part of the problem is that we are not quite sure what we are looking for. We do not even have an agreed language for talking about the relation between brains and experiences. Depending on the neuroscientist, brain events are 'associated with', 'caused by', 'related to', or just plain 'are' conscious states. The core of the difficulty is clear. A change in the state of my brain may be experienced by me as a change in the appearance of the Necker cube, but will be experienced by a neuroscientist as a change in the firing rate of cells in my temporal lobe. Feeble attempts have been made by philosophers to say that this is no different from describing the same planet Venus as the 'Morning Star' and the 'Evening Star', but they add little to our understanding. We almost certainly need to think about consciousness and the brain in an entirely new way, but the organ holding us up is the very one we are trying to understand. Under the force of natural selection, the brain has evolved a way of thinking about itself and its relation to the outside world that has served it well; but science will have to advance beyond this common-sense picture if it wants to make progress; and two millennia of philosophical failure show that it will not do so within the limits of ordinary language.

This book has *not* explained how nerve cells give rise to conscious experience, but it has argued that the brain is a collection of specialised machines, much more like old-fashioned analogue computers than the modern digital computer with its central processor. Many of these analogue engines rely on maps. Space is not represented in the brain in an abstract way, but by the spatial layout of nerve cells and their connections.

Does it matter what kind of computer the brain is? There are two extreme views about the relation between structure and function in the brain. The view called 'strong AI' holds that it does not matter whether the brain is made of nerve cells or blue cheese; and it does not matter either whether it does its computations using numbers or analogue computers. Any machine that acts in an intelligent way has artificial intelligence. Any machine that can interpret images as we do is having visual perceptions; and so on. 'Strong AI' theorists use the work of Alan Turing to argue that the distinction between analogue and digital computing is trivial. Any analogue computer can be simulated by a digital computer. Kelvin's tide computer with its wheels and pulleys can be reproduced by a digital computer using the mathematics of the 'Fast Fourier Transform'. Bill Phillips' hydraulic model of the economy was supplanted years ago by more sophisticated numerical models in digital computers. Most neural network models of human cognition have never existed outside of simulations on a digital computer. The case that digital computers can simulate any computing machine is overwhelming, both in theory and in practice.

Against this, opponents of 'strong AI' say that a digital computer is merely a number cruncher, programmed by a human operator to simulate something else. The digital computer is a glorified adding machine, which probably has no experiences at all; or if it does have any, they are experiences as remote from anything we can imagine as the thoughts of a hydrogen atom. The computer itself cannot possibly know what it is simulating, and it has no idea what its output means. It requires the brain of the person who programmed the computer to know what the calculations mean. A computer simulating global weather patterns may just possibly be having some sort of experiences, but there is no reason at all to suppose that these experiences are about the weather. A computer analysing the pixels of an image does not know that it is looking at an image rather than a matrix of numbers. The computer model of weather is just a series of mathematical equations. If we think that these equations are 'experiences', why aren't equations conscious when written on a piece of paper? Confusing numbers with reality is no better than a particularly loopy form of Platonism.

Everything useful that can be said about this problem in the present feeble state of our knowledge probably has been said, and it is tempting to agree on this point at least with the gloomy French philosopher: 'It's all been said before.' Some things are on common ground. We can all probably agree that there is a big problem in attributing conscious experiences to a computer quietly humming away to itself in a corner. What, indeed, would those experiences be about? The Abbé de Condillac imagined a human statue in a similar position, and concluded that the statue would have to move about the world before it experienced that world as we do. At the other extreme, we can all agree that a machine that walks, talks and blushes as we do is having human experiences; after all, mating couples make thousands of such machines every minute, and they are admitted to the human race without question. A machine that moves around the world and interacts with it can check its internal models against incoming data. This gets around the problem of meaning: the meaning of the model is in the world outside, not in the machine. There is no longer any need for an operator to program the machine and interpret its output; but engaging with the world has its price, as we all discover. There are rules to be obeyed. The machine that enters the real world has at some stage to abandon its numerical codes and obey the real rules of space and time. Its internal models cannot just be the Bellman's 'arbitrary signs'. I am suggesting that any really effective machine that moves about in its environment and interacts with it will have a strong analogue computing element, like our brain. Time will tell. We may, as the AI theorist hopes, understand our minds one day without understanding the machinery of the brain. But I don't think so.

Notes

Preface

The prize for the worst poem about Science has yet to be awarded.
For the Royal Society verse see Erich Heller (1971) *The Disinherited Mind* (Cambridge: Bowes & Bowes). For the bear and mackerel see Steve Jones *Almost Like a Whale: 'The Origin of Species Updated'* (Anchor: Transworld Publishers). For the 'Mazy Course': J. Millott Severn *'Phrenology: The Language of the Mental Faculties'*, published by the author, 20 Middle Street Brighton, England. The phreonolgist's son Dr Adolph Gladstone Millott Severn was a medical man and an important collector of the works of Aubrey Beardsley.

Neuroscientists for obvious reasons tend to favour the first view, but it is a notoriously difficult theory to sell to our brains.
The logical reasons why a brain might be puzzled by its own experiences are explored by Hofststadter, D. & Dennett, D. (1981) *The Mind's I: Fantasies and Reflections on Self and Soul*, Sussex: Harvester Press. The problem has been given an evolutionary spin by asking why consciousness has evolved in addition to brains. The question assumes dualism as its premise. A version asks how we would recognise a 'zombie' who had brain states like ours but no awareness. Perhaps there are zombies here amongst us, hosting chat shows on TV or presenting Fox News. An attempt to organise a conference for zombies to discuss the problem of consciousness was a complete success, like the first meeting of the International Anarchists Association. No one turned up.

1: Murder on the Highway

But should a photographic image be admissible as evidence in Court of Law?
For the history of this legal argument see the Web site http://chnm.gmu.aq/photos/essay/4.htm, from which the quotations are taken. For optograms, I am indebted to an article by Arthur B. Evans 'Optograms and Fiction' (http://jv.gilead.org.il/evans/optogram.html) and to John Mollon for bringing the Web site to my attention. The descriptions of Kühne's experiments in Evans' article are in turn based on the article 'Eye and Camera' (1976) by George Wald.

The eye does indeed form an image on the retina, but its purpose is not as obvious as that of an image in a camera.

The experiment of blur adaptation was reported by Webster, M. A., Georgeson, M. A. & Webster, S. M. (2002) 'Neural adjustments to image blur', *Nat. Neurosci.*, 5, 839–42. For an argument that we are not normally conscious of the blur of moving objects, for the same reason, see Burr, D. C. & Morgan, M. J. (1997), Motion deblurring in human vision. *Proc. Roy. Soc. Lond.*, 264B, 431–6.

This becomes cruelly obvious with advancing age, and deterioration of vision is usually our first intimation of mortality.
For pinholes see *http://www.pinholes.com*

There is nothing inherently defective about the moderately myopic eye: it is simply adapted to a different viewing distance from the so-called normal eye.
Wallman, J. & Adams, J. I. (1987), 'Developmental aspects of experimental myopia in chicks: susceptibility, recovery and relation to emmetropization', *Vision Res.*, 27(7), 1139–63.

The original purpose of forming an image in the eye may have been to increase the amount of light falling on the photoreceptors. . .
For the calculation of a 2 per cent difference at threshold see Morgan, M. J. & Aiba, T. S. (1987) 'Vernier acuity predicted from changes in the light distribution of the retinal image', *Spatial Vision*, 1, 151–171. For a general review of the limits to the vision of objects, Morgan M. J. (1990) Hyperacuity, in *Spatial Vision* (ed. M. Regan). London: Macmillan.

Berkeley's solution was to say that experience comes to our aid and teaches us to associate visual impressions with the true properties of objects. . .Visual sensations have no resemblance to the properties of objects. They are entirely arbitrary symbols like the words in a language. . .
De Selby held to almost exactly the contrary theory. (For the views of this philosopher on Motion see chapter 5). He regarded words as resembling the visual qualities of the objects they denoted. It was 'not entirely a coincidence' that the words 'black' and 'noir' have a certain 'dead' and 'heavy' quality. The elegant flight of the eponymous insect is conveyed both by 'butterfly' and by 'papillon', and even by 'Schmetterling'. Even the mild Leclerc was moved to remark that on this occasion the savant seemed to have confused Entomology and Etymology. De Selby's theories of the origin of language give a useful clue to his state of mind on this occasion. He denied the 'Anglo-Saxon' theory that language evolved for the giving of orders, and preferred the 'Celtic' alternative that it was for singing and deception.

There is both good and bad news from modern neuroscience for Berkeley's theory of vision. . .True, Descartes had earlier scorned the idea that the eye sends little images into the brain. . .
'Although this little picture (sc the retinal image) still retains some resemblance to the objects from which it originates, as it passes to the back of the head, we should not fall into the error of thinking that it is by the means of this resemblance that we see the objects; for there is not another set of eyes in the head with which we could see these images. Rather, Nature has determined that we should experience certain sensations when the movements from which these images are composed, act directly on our mind

through its link with the body.' (Quoted by Merleau-Ponty from the *Dioptrique* in *La Structure du Comportement*, Paris: Presses Universitaires, 1967, p. 206).

Just as endlessly repeated was the story of the man, blind from birth.
There was an actual case, described by Cheselden, of a young man operated on for the removal of cataract. The patient behaved impeccably according to empiricist theories. At first he saw little, but after picking up a cat, famously remarked 'So Puss! I shall know you again.' The account has to be taken with a pinch of salt. For the debate on recovery from congenital blindness see Morgan, M. J. (1977), *Molyneux's Question: vision, touch and the philosophy of perception* (Cambridge University Press).

It is no coincidence that the philosophers of the Enlightenment chose blindness as one of their main metaphors for fighting the ecclesiastical and civil authorities...John Locke's Treatise of Civil Government *was as familiar as the Bible to the colonists of the American Revolution.*
Attributed to the American Historian E.S. Morgan by James White *The Origins of Modern Europe*, London: John Murray, 1964, p. 356.

Some may therefore sympathise with the ideology behind Condillac's statue – but that does make it a correct account of vision.
The pressure-phosphere experiment was reported by Sclodtmann, W. (1902) 'Ein Betrag zur Lehre von der optischen Localisation bei Blindgeborene', *Archiv. f. Ophthalmologie*, 54, 256–67. I thank Mitch Glickstein for telling me about this experiment and for allowing me to consult his handwritten translation. For re-growth of the frog optic nerve see Sperry, R.W. (1959), 'The growth of nerve circuits', *Scientific American* 201:68–75.

The tough question here is whether Stratton and Kohler had really learned to see the world 'the right way up'.
See Wade, N. (2000), 'An upright man', *Perception*, 29, 253–7. For Mirrors in general see Richard Gregory's *Mirrors in Mind*, London: Penguin. The classic experiment on pointing to an unseen sound source was done by Harris, C. S. (1963) 'Adaptation to displaced vision: visual, motor or proprioceptive change?' *Science*, 140, 812–13.

The right-hand image of a famous face in figure 1.3 looks grotesque...
See Thompson, P. (1980) 'Margaret Thatcher: a new illusion.' *Perception* 9:483–4

This experiment has not been done, but a similar one has.
Linden, D. E. et al (1999) 'The myth of upright vision. A psychophysical and functional imaging study of adaptation to inverting spectacles.' *Perception*, 28(4), 469–81.

2: Conventional Signs

Wyld's 1815 'Chart of Civilisations' colours countries.
See 'Lie of the Land: the secret life of maps', from the 2001–2002 Exhibition at the British Library (edited by April Carluuci and Peter Barber and published by the British Library, 2001).

The uselessness of a map that is merely an image is also the theme of a story in Borges and Casares' Extraordinary Tales.

'Exactitude' tells of an Empire in which the Schools of Cartography become so obsessed with accuracy that they produced, first of all, maps of a province the size of a City and finally, a map of the Kingdom which corresponded to the whole Kingdom point for point. There are echoes here of the life-work of Pierre Menard, which consisted of the ninth and thirty-eighth chapter of Part One of *Don Quixote* and a fragment of the twenty-second chapter – recreated *de novo* word for word.

Herman Lotze taught in Göttingen and his book 'Medical Psychology' was published in 1852.
Lotze thought he was applying the philosophy of Immanuel Kant to the perception of space. In fact, Kant would almost certainly have called Lotze's efforts 'a labour lost'. Kant did not think that space was an arbitrary representation like a smell. It is true that he muddies the waters in places by seeming to say that Space and Time are, like colours, just representations of the unknowable. He even says that Space and Time are only representations of the human mind, and 'not necessarily shared in by every being'. (*General Observations on Transcendental Aesthetic*) seeming to make them arbitrary features of a purely human cognition. For an account of the 'Two Faces of the Critique' see Strawson, P. F. *'The Bounds of Sense'* (1966, London: Methuen). Kant accepted that Space and Time were different from colours, tones and smells. He said that colour could be 'empirically deduced' from Space and Time, but that Space and Time could allow only a 'Transcendental Deduction'. A transcendental deduction refers to an explanation transcending the senses altogether. The ambitious aim of the *Critique of Pure Reason* is to show that any conscious mind whatsoever would have to experience space and time. It is therefore inevitable that our explanations of the world use a spatio-temporal language. If we want a scientific theory of how the brain represents space, it is going to have to be a spatial theory, according to Kant.

A celebrated paper entitled 'What the frog's eye tells the frog's brain'...
Lettvin, J. Y., Maturana, R. R., McCulloch, W. S. & Pitts, W. H. (1959) 'What the frog's eye tells the frog's brain.' *Proc. Inst. Rad. Eng.*, 47, 1940–51. The term 'receptive field' was coined by Hartline, who discovered lateral inhibition in the eye of the horseshoe crab. The 'centre-surround' organisation of receptive fields in the frog retina was discovered independently by Horace Barlow and Stephen Kuffler.

Graded molecules in the retina and tectum are not the only signposts available.
A protein signpost called 'Roundabout' has the responsibility of directing traffic at the midline. See Tear, G. (2001) 'A new code for axons', *Nature*, 409, 472–3.

The neighbourhood rule would not necessarily work in a different environment from our own.
See Wong, R. (1999) 'Retinal waves and visual development.' *Annu. Rev. Neurosci.*, 22–9.

A map is no good if it cannot be read.
For the story of the crate see Jones, R. V. (1988) *Most Secret War*, Ware: Wordsworth Editions Ltd.

Amphibians do indeed catch their prey without the help of this useless non-spatial entrepreneur.

This account has obviously been much simplified. The picture is complicated by the fact that amphibians have a second visual pathway, more analogous to the largest visual pathway in humans, going to the forebrain via the thalamus. This pathway can control and inhibit prey-catching behaviour. For more detail see Ewert, J-P and Arbib, M. A. (eds.), *Visuomotor Coordination: Amphibians, Comparisons, Models and Robots* (1989) Plenum Press, and review articles by Cervantes-Pérez, F. 'Visuomotor coordination in Frogs and Toads' and G. Manteufel 'Visuomotor coordination in salamanders' in Arbib, M. A. (ed.), 1995, *The Handbook of Brain Theory and Neural Networks*, Bradford Books/The MIT Press.

3: 'The long-agitated question'

The defeat of the Russians at Port Arthur in 1904 was one of the seismic events of the 20th Century.

I am indebted to Manfred Fahle and Mitch Glickstein for giving me a copy of their translation of Inouye's work from the original German (special supplement to the journal *Brain*, 123, 2000) and for discussing it with me.

If we look at a scene first through one eye and then through the other, we shall find that the two views are very similar.

De Selby's dislike of Newton (and in particular of his 'reductionist' theory of colour) led the savant to a characteristically original theory about the connection between the eyes, which need not detain us long. Basing his ideas on the 'well known case' in which the optogram of a murderer was imprinted in the eye of a victim *wearing an eye patch*, de Selby proposed that the image in one eye is always copied directly to the retina of the other by a 'collateral pathway'. The savant's theory of binocular fusion was the cause of the celebrated 'Copenhagen dispute' about what Nelson really saw through his telescope at the eponymous naval battle. Du Garbandier thought little of de Selby's theory of binocular vision. It reminded him, he said, of the Oxford professor who was observed pumping up the rear tyre of his bicycle. 'What? Do they not communicate?' was his response when a passer-by helpfully pointed out that it was in fact the front tyre that was flat.

How Newton arrived at this theory, no one knows; but his inspired guess was supported in 1824 by the English physician and scientist William Hyde Wollaston.

See 'On semi-decussation of the Optic Nerves', *Phil. Trans. Roy. Soc.* 114, (1824), 222–31.

In Gennari's stripe all the nerve cells are driven either from the left eye or the right.

For Gennari's history see Mitchell Glickstein 'The Discovery of the Visual Cortex', *Scientific American*, 1988,118–27

Why are there so many different maps in the brain, instead of a single master map?

The numbers of nerve cells are taken from Shepherd G. M. & Koch, C. (1990) 'Introduction to synaptic circuits' in Shepherd, G. M. (ed.) *The synaptic organisation of the brain*, Oxford University Press.

4: Cyclopean Vision

'Neither reply nor pity came from him.'
Lines 287–290 of the *Odyssey*, translated by Robert Fitzgerald, 1988, London: The Harvill Press. We cannot be sure that the *Odyssey* was first told by Homer, but if not by Homer, the poem was certainly created by another blind scholar of the same name. De Selby argues that Homer's listeners probably knew many cases of soldiers who had lost an eye in battle yet who could still fight effectively. In his seminal review of the literature, de Selby rightly concluded that we do not need two eyes to see the world in three dimensions. Nor, according to the fossil record, do other animals. The legend of Cyclops was based on the discovery by the ancient Greeks of real fossils with a gigantic hole in the middle of their forehead, 'of which creature we may say that it was probably not a rhinoceros, but little more' (de Selby, *Cyclopean Vision*, p. 1332). De Selby reviews several interesting Darwinian theories about the origin of the second eye: the 'Symmetry' theory according to which two eyes are better than one because they allow females to choose the most symmetrical mate; the not-unrelated 'Disadvantage' theory which states that females prefer mates who have faced up to the challenge of combining images from the two eyes; and the 'Black Jack' theory, whose central conjecture is that if we lose one eye, it is useful to have another so that we may distinguish sheep from sailors wearing fleeces (*Mutiny on the Beagle*, chapter 12).

The idea that we need two eyes to see the world in three dimensions is a delusion.
I have stated the argument that the eye is not a rangefinder in an extreme form, which should be qualified. Although our brain cannot measure the angle between the eyes with precision from the muscular effort involved, Mayhew & Longuet-Higgins have shown that the angle can be determined from differences in the images between the two eyes. Specifically, if three points do not lie on the same retinal meridian, the 'viewing parameters' of convergence distance and angle of eccentric gaze can be derived from the horizontal and vertical differences between the positions of the points in the two eyes (horizontal and vertical disparities). See Mayhew, J. & Longuet-Higgins, H. C. (1982) 'A computational model of binocular depth perception.' *Nature*, 297, 376–8, and the extended discussion of the role of vertical disparities in Howard, I. P. & Rogers, B. J. (1995) *Binocular Vision and Stereopsis*. Oxford: Oxford University Press. pp. 283–92. A device called the 'telestereoscope' proves the importance of binocular convergence angle for computing range. Like a long-base rangefinder (that in *'Bismarck'* had a base of 9 metres) the telestereoscope uses mirrors to increase the virtual distance between the two eyes. This alters the normal relation between convergence angle and range, and observers using a telestereoscope make errors when reaching for objects. However, these errors disappear with practice, showing that observers can recalibrate the distance between their eyes (see Howard & Rogers, op cit.).

In fact, we do not need two eyes at all to see the third dimension.
'The Five Senses' is part of the collection of still-lifes in the Musée des Beaux Arts. The catalogue is in *Natures Mortes*, Édition des musées de la Ville, Strasbourg, 1964. One assumes that Vision is indicated by a member of the canine persuasion (the small black object with a tail, by the river) because it is in the distance, and vision is the distance sense.

The relationship between shadows and shape is subtle, and not always intuitively obvious.

For a different view on the Signorelli example see Cavanagh, P. (1999) 'Pictorial art and illusion' in R. A. Wilson & F. C. Keil, (eds.) *MIT Encylopaedia of Cognitive Science*, MIT Press. I am grateful to Chris McManus for pointing out to me that the shadows must meet at the torso. An excellent book on shadows is Baxandall, M. *'Shadows and the Enlightenment'* (1995) New Haven: Yale University Press.

Atmospheric perspective
Bishop Berkeley was one of several to invoke atmospheric effects to explain the harvest moon illusion. He echoes de Selby in implicating 'black air' as the cause of the illusion: 'Further, the air being variously impregnated, sometimes more and sometimes less, with vapours and exhalations fitted to retund and intercept the rays of light, it follows that the appearance of the horizontal moon hath not always an equal faintness, and by consequence that luminary, though in the very same situation, is at one time judged greater than at another' but stops just short of blaming the accumulation of black air on the avariciousness of irresponsible industrialists. As nearly always happens with new inventions, the stereoscope was rapidly followed by claims that it had been discovered before. For an entertaining account of the Wheatstone–Brewster controversy see Wade, N. J. (2002). Charles Wheatstone (1802–1875). *Perception*, 31, 265–72.

To discover another advantage of binocular vision, try picking blackberries with one eye closed.
Morgan, M. J. (1989). 'Vision of solid objects', *Nature*, 339, 101–03. For an experiment showing that two eyes are better than one see Servos, P., Goodale, M. A. & Jakobson, L. S. (1992) 'The role of binocular vision in prehension: a kinematic analysis.' *Vision Res.*, 32(8), 1513–21.

Another example is 'shape from shading'.
The shading-sensitive nerve cells are described by Connor, C. E. (2001) 'Visual Perception: Sunny Side Up', *Curr. Biol.*, 11, R776–R778. The cells combining texture and disparity are in the caudal intraparietal sulcus and were described by Tsutsui, K. I. et al. (2002) 'Neural correlates for perception of 3D surface orientation from texture gradients', *Science*, 298, 409. For comment see Conner, C. E. (2002) 'Reconstructing a 3D world', *Science*, 298, 376–7.

There is a final twist in the story of binocular vision.
For the 'empty Rhine' see Babbington-Smith, B. (1977). 'A wartime anticipation of random-dot stereograms', *Perception*, 6, 233–4. For the invention of random-dot stereograms see Julesz, B. (1971) *Foundations of Cyclopean Perception*, Chicago: University of Chicago Press; and Howard, I. P. & Rogers, B. J. (1995) *Binocular Vision and Stereopsis*, Oxford: Oxford University Press. For a review of the physiology of binocular stereopsis see DeAngelis, G. C. (2000) 'Seeing in three dimensions: the neurophysiology of stereopsis', *Trends in Cognitive Sciences*, 4, 80–90.

Computer simulations show that this simple analogue computation solves the random-dot problem particularly efficiently if combined with the other two rules described earlier.
For the models see Marr, D. & Poggio, T. (1976) 'Cooperative computation of stereo disparity', *Science*, 194, 283–7; Marr, D. & Poggio, T. (1979) 'A computational theory of human stereo vision', *Proc. R. Soc. Lond.* B, 204, 301–28. For the evidence that parallax-

tuned nerve neurones cluster in V5/MT see DeAngelis, G. C. (2000) 'Seeing in three dimensions: the neurophysiology of stereopsis', *Trends in Cognitive Sciences*, 4, 80–90.

5: 'Objects moving are not impressed'

Persistence of vision is not a sufficient explanation of motion.
The modern version of Exner's motion detector is called the 'Reichardt detector', after the German physiologist who, with Hassenstein, described the basic mechanism in the beetle *Chlorophanus*. For references see Morgan, M. J. & Chubb, C. (1999) 'Contrast facilitation in motion detection: evidence for a Reichardt detector in human vision', *Vision Res.*, 39, 4217–4131.

A simple experiment to show that motion is not perceived as a series of frames is shown in Figure 5.2.
For details and discussion of this experiment see (1) Burr, D. C. (1979) 'Acuity for apparent vernier offset', *Vision Res.*, 19, 835–7. (2) Morgan, M. (1980) 'Analogue models of motion perception', *Phil. Trans. R. Soc. Ser. B.* (3) Morgan, M. J.(1976) 'Pulfrich effect and the filling in of apparent motion', *Perception*, 5, 187–95.

Our simple-minded mechanisms are also fooled by the 'waterfall effect'.
A special issue of the journal *Perception* (1994, 23, 1107–1264) was devoted to the motion after-effect. For an illustration of the waterfall effect itself see: http://www.biols.susx.ac.uk/home.George – Mather/Motion/MAE.HTML. For a selection of articles on the mechanisms of adaptation and the motion after-effect see: (1) Barlow, H. & Földiák, P. (1989) 'Adaptation and decorrelation in the cortex' in R. Darbin & C. Miall & G. Mitchison (eds.), *The Computing Neuron*, Wesley Publishers Ltd.; (2) Carlson, V. R. (1962) 'Adaptation in the perception of visual velocity', *J. Exp. Psychol*, 64, 192–7; (3) Harris, R. A., O'Carroll, D. C., & Laughlin, S. B. (1999) 'Adaptation and the temporal delay filter of fly motion detectors', *Vision Res.*, 39(16), 2603–13; (4) Mather, G., Anstis, S., & Verstraten, F., *The Motion Aftereffect*,Cambridge, Mass.: MIT Press; (5) Rapoport, J. (1964) 'Adaptation in the perception of rotary motion', *Journal of Experimental Psychology*, 67, 263–7.

Single 'coincidence detectors' analyse only a small area of the retinal image.
The problems that arise from not seeing the big picture are evident when looking at motion through a narrow aperture. An everyday example is the 'barber pole' effect. (The white and red bands of the barber pole were the insignia of the Guild of Barber-Surgeons). The pole rotates around a horizontal axis and the true movement of the stripes is thus vertical to the line of sight of the eye. But most of the time we perceive the movement of the stripes *along* the pole. From the point of view of a small analogue motion detector tilted in the same direction as the stripes, the movement is indistinguishable from that of a horizontally-moving stripe. In this case, the brain is prevented from getting the big picture because there is nothing to give the true direction of movement.

A neurological patient studied in Munich has damage to the higher centres for motion perception.
See Hess, R. H., Baker, C. L. & Zihl, J. (1989) 'The "motion-blind" patient: low level spatial and temporal filters', *Journal Neurosci.*, 9, 1628–40; Zihl, J., Cramon, D., & Mai,

N. (1983) 'Selective disturbance of movement vision after bilateral brain damage', *Brain*, 106, 313–40.

Motion perception depends on specialised mechanisms in the brain, as does 'Cyclopean Vision.'
For the 'snowstorm' illusion see: Morgan, M. J., & Fahle, M. (2000) 'Motion-stereo mechanisms sensitive to inter-ocular phase', *Vision Res.*, 40, 1667–75.

6: 'Actual dynamical models of things'

A good Web site on Analogue computers is:
http://dcoward.best.vwh.net/analog/analog1.htm
Lord Kelvin used a computer to predict the movement of water, but we can just as easily reverse the process and use water as a computer. For Phillips' water computer see Pain (2000) 'A liquid computer', *New Scientist*, 9 December, and the Science Museum Gallery Guide on the Web http://www.sciencemuseum.org.uk/galleryguide/E2221.asp

Arthur Pollen had an unusual background for an inventor.
Pollen's papers are held in the Churchill Archive at Cambridge. My account is based on the following sources: Sumida, J. (1984a) *In Defence of Naval Supremacy*, Boston: Unwin Hyman; Sumida, J. (1984b) *The Pollen Papers*, published by George Allen & Unwin for the Naval Records Society.; Brooks, J. (2001) 'Fire control for British Dreadnoughts', Unpublished Ph.D. thesis, Department of War Studies, King's College London. For Hannibal Choate Ford, see Clymer, A. B. (1993) 'The Mechanical Analog Computers of Hannibal Ford and William Newell', *IEEE Annals of the History of Computing*, 15, 19–34.

Almon B. Strowger was an undertaker with a problem.
http://www.strowger.com/history.html.
For the history of switching: http://www/seg.co.uk/telecomm/automat1.htm. For more on Claude Shannon: http://www.nyu.edu/pages/linguistics/courses/v610003/shan.html

7: Machines that Learn

Engineers might never have tried to solve such a difficult problem if not encouraged by the fact that simple brains had solved it first.
For the pigeon experiment see Morgan, M. J. et al (1976) 'Pigeons learn the concept of an "A"', *Perception*, 5, 57–66.

The high girders of the Tay Bridge would not have blown down...
See Rolt, L. T. C., *Red for Danger*, Pan Books (1986)

A Perceptron-like switching circuit was demonstrated at a 1960 convention of the Institute of Radio Engineers in New York City.
Widrow, B., & Hoff, M. (1960) 'Adaptive switching circuits', *IRE Wescon Convention Record* (NY:IRE) pp. 96–104.

When a soap bubble is drawn out between two or more rings it takes on a complicated shape, very difficult to predict in advance.

Hopfield, J. J. (1982) 'Neural networks and physical systems with emergent collective computational abilities', *Proc. Natl. Acad. Sci. USA*, 79, 2554–8.

One day, artificial neural networks could make good the damage to real nervous systems.
For the neurobiotic rat see Chapin, J. K. et al. (1999) 'Real-time control of a robot arm using simultaneously recorded neurons in the motor cortex', *Nat. Neurosci.*, 27, 664–70

8: Controlled Hallucination

'Perception is nothing more than successful hallucination'
Clowes, M. (1971) 'On seeing things', *Artificial Intelligence*, 2, 79–112

The Reverend Bayes was born in London.
For a statement of Bayes' Theorem and its significance see Dayan, P. & Abbott, L. F. (2001) *Theoretical Neuroscience*, Cambridge Mass.: MIT Press, p. 88.

For example, why does a lump of coal look black?
For a recent attempt to apply Bayesian reasoning to brightness perception see Purves, D. & Lotto, B. (2003) *Why We See What We Do*, Sinauer Associates.

Models of this kind are called 'generative models,' because they try to generate the data.
I first heard the harbour analogy from Al Bregmann of McGill University. For a brief review of generative models and further references see Hinton, G. (2000) 'Computation by neural networks', *Nature Neuroscience Supplement*, 3,1170. For the deep relation between factor analysis, PCA, and other generative models see Roweis, S. & Ghahramani, Z. (1999) 'A unifying review of linear Gaussian Models', *Neural Computation*,11, 305–45.

Computers use generative models for translating human speech into written words.
See Hinton, G. (2000) 'Computation by neural networks', *Nature Neuroscience Supplement*, 3,1170.

If perceptions are internal models, we should be able to experience them without images on the retina.
Coleridge wrote: 'In the summer of the year 1797, the Author, then in ill health, had returned to a lonely farm-house between Porlock and Lindon, on the Exmoor confines of Somerset and Devonshire. In consequence of a slight indisposition, an anodyne had been prescribed, from the effects of which he fell asleep in his chair at the moment when he was reading the following sentence, or words of the same substance, in Purchas's Pilgrimage "Here the Khan Kubla commanded a palace to be built, and a stately garden thereunto."' (*Poems*, Selected and Edited by John Beer, Everyman's Library, reprinted 1982).

Laughing gas, ether, laudanum and hashish were all regularly and legally used in 19th Century 'frolics.'
See Chapter 8 of *The Forbidden Game* by Brian Aldiss (NY: Charles Scribner, 1975).

9: The Babel Library of Icons

In his story 'The Library of Babel' . . .
Borges, J. L. (1962) 'The Library of Babel', in *Fictions* Anthony Kerrigan, (ed.) London: John Calder.

The problem with looking at an image is that we instantly perceive its meaning (if it has one) rather than its pixels.
For a variety of image landscapes see Watt, R. J. (1991) *Understanding Vision*, Academic Press.

Once we get into the habit of thinking about images as landscapes, we can begin to manipulate them.
In arithmetical terms, blurring is accomplished by replacing each pixel with the average of its own value and that of the pixels in a neighbourhood around it. The larger the neighbourhood, the more severe the blurring.

If images contain these large-scale structures, a pixel-by-pixel description becomes unnecessary, or in grammatical terms 'redundant.'
For image compression algorithms in general see Gonzalez, R. C. & Woods, R. E. (1993) *Digital Image Processing*, Addison Wesley. Algorithms are divided into 'lossy', which lose information, and 'non-lossy' in which all the information is retained, but in a compressed form.

The cat in Figure 9.4.1 is easily recognised from its abstract outline drawing.
For the 'primal sketch' see David Marr's book *Vision*. David Marr was a seminal and controversial figure in the theory of vision. After studying Mathematics at Cambridge he became interested in physiology and developed a formal model of the relation between structure and function of the cerebellum. After moving to MIT he became interested in Machine Vision and developed, with Tomaso Poggio the idea that it is useless to start simulating vision on a computer without having a clear theory of vision in the first place. By a 'computational theory of vision' Marr and Poggio meant, first of all, a clear understanding of the physical nature of images and the abstract rules that could be followed to get back from images to what is 'out here'. Only then would it be profitable to produce a model of how the brain carried out this process with real nerve cells.

An early pioneer in using sketches to transmit information across the telegraph was Francis Galton.
Galton, F. (1910) Numeralised profiles for classification and recognition, *Nature*, 83,127–30.

The brain's description of texture begins in primary visual cortex.
Mathematically, the 'striped receptive fields' are called 'Gabor patches', after Dennis Gabor. There is a very large literature on the use of Gabor functions for image analysis. A particularly clear and readable essay is by Robson, J. (1980) 'Neural Images', in C. S. Harris (ed.), *The Physiological Basis of Spatial Vision, Visual Coding and Adaptability*, Hillsdale, N. J.: Earlbaum, pp177–214.. Neural networks have discovered receptive fields like Gabor functions by themselves when trained with natural images: see Olshausen, B. A. & Field, D. J. (1986) 'Emergence of simple-cell receptive field properties by learning a spare code for natural images', *Nature*, 381, 607–9.

Gabor receptive fields may be good at finding ridges and cliffs in image landscapes, but only in their own small patch of the image.
They do this particularly convincingly when used to construct a map of 'local energy'. See Morrone, C. & Burr, D. (1990) 'Feature detection in human vision: a phase-dependent energy model', *Proc. Roy. Soc. B.*, 235, 221–45.

The highest-ranking members of the hierarchy discovered so far are in the temporal lobe of the monkey.
Gross, C. G., Rocha-Miranda, C. E., & Bender, D. B. (1972) 'Visual Properties of neurons in inferotemporal cortex of the macaque', *J. Neurophysiol.*, 35, 96–111. A common objection to single cell recording at the time was that it cannot be expected to tell us anything very interesting. What could the activity of one cell amongst thousands of millions possibly tell us about the working of the brain as a whole? After all, it was objected, if we stuck a small electrode into the innards of a digital computer, we would learn nothing about what program the machine was running. Even recording from many cells at once by electrodes on the surface of the scalp was equally pointless, like trying to learn French by recording sound signals from a high-flying aircraft over Paris. And for the final stupidity, what about recording from the brain when the animal was under anaesthesia: this is like recording from a computer when it is turned off! All this just goes to show how misleading logical analogies can be, particularly those based on brains and digital computers. In reality, signals from certain cells in the lower part of the temporal lobe of the monkey turned out to be highly informative. For columns of feature cells see Fujita I., Tanaka K., Ito M., & Cheng, K. (1992) 'Columns for visual features of objects in monkey inferotemporal cortex', *Nature*, 360, 343–6.; Tanaka, K. (1996) 'Inferotemporal cortex and object vision', *Annual Review of Neuroscience*,19,109–39.

The late Maurice Bowra liked to confuse people by saying 'I know your name, but I can't remember your face.'
For the theory of 'face recognition units' see Bruce V., Burton A. M., & Craw, I. (1992) 'Modelling face recognition', *Phil. Trans .R. Soc. Lond.*, 335,121–8. For references on prosopagnosia and for the fMRI experiment on developmental prosopagnosics see a recent paper by Hadjikhani, N. & De Gelder, B. (2002) 'Neural basis of Prosopagnosia: An fMRI study', *Human Brain Mapping*,16,176–82. For references to farmers, sheep and birds see McNeil, J., & Warrington, E. K. (1993) 'Prosopagnosia: a face-specific disorder', *Quarterly Journal of Experimental Psychology*, A46, 1–10.; Bornstein, B. (1963) 'Prosopagnosia', in L. Helpern (ed.) *Problems of Dynamic Neurology*, Jerusalem: Hadessah Medical Organization.

Eigenfaces can be used to make caricatures.
The idea behind 'Principal Component Analysis' is to find a space in which the faces are spread as evenly as possible, like currants in a well-mixed cake, rather than like the stars in the Universe, which cluster into Galaxies. The input to a computer program that does PCA is a set of face images, each containing the same number of pixels. The output is another set of images, the same size as the original, containing face-like images, but not the original set. For reasons of mathematical terminology that need not concern us here, the output images are called 'Eigenfaces.' We can guarantee that any individual set of faces in original set can be synthesised by adding together the Eigenfaces in different proportions. So far, we can synthesise 'n' faces from 'n' Eigenfaces. No economy has been achieved. But it turns out that most of the Eigenfaces add little to the synthesis. They

are concerned with petty detail, which we do not need for face recognition. Only ten or so Eigenfaces are needed to produce recognisable versions of the original. The most important Eigenface is the average image, as defined by Galton. Not unnaturally, this always appears as the most important ingredient in the image cake. We now need only a small set of numbers to describe any individual face, each number representing the strength of a particular Eigenface in the mixture. For example, if we used 5 Eigenfaces and an individual just happened to have a face identical to the average face, he or she would get the code 1 0 0 0 0; another individual might be 0.95 0.1 0.2 0.3 0.1; and so on. If the original images are 256 x 256 pixels we have achieved the extraordinary economy of reducing a space of 256 x 256 dimensions in Pixelese to only 5 dimensions in a 'face space'. This is much better even than Galton's four-dimensional space for face profiles. For the original paper on Eigenfaces see: Turk, M. A. & Pentland, A. P. (1991) 'Face recognition using Eigenfaces', *IEEE*, 586–91. The experiment on 'anti-faces' was done with two faces called 'Adam' and 'Anti-Adam' and computer-generated intermediates by Leopold, D. A. et al (2001) 'Prototype-references shape encoding revealed by high-level after-effects', *Nature Neuroscience*, 4, 89--94.

10: 'Whirling madly through the darkness'

For reviews of frames of reference see Rock, I. (1966) *The Nature of Perceptual Adaptation* (Basic Books), and Howard, I. P. & Templeton, W. B. (1966) *Human Spatial Orientation* (Wiley).

The book from which these two examples are taken goes on to give 22 properties of physical space in all.
Ian Hinckfuss (1975) *The Existence of Space and Time*, Oxford: Clarendon Press, Chapter 2.

In physical space, an object remains the same object when it is rotated. Not so for us.
'Mental rotation' was first described by Roger Shepard and his colleagues, and a review of their work will be found in Shepard, R. N. & Cooper, L. A. (1982) *Mental Images and Their Transformations*, Cambridge, Mass.: MIT Press. The phenomenon can be observed with shapes as simple as the letters of the alphabet. Ask yourself whether the letter 'p' is a rotated version of a 'd' or a 'b'? Shepard & Metzler used perspective views of three-dimensional 'Lego' shapes. They then halted their observers part-way through the mental rotation process and got them to describe the figure they were imagining (Shepard, R. N. & Meltzer, J. (1971) 'Mental rotation of three-dimensional objects', *Science*, 171, 701–3). For further links see: http://Cognet.mit.edu/Mitecs/Entry/tarr.html

Sometimes a reference frame changes spontaneously, and we perceive a figure changing its orientation without any physical change in the image.
Perceptually-reversing figures tell us that there is a distinction between an image (as a physical object) and seeing an image *as* something. Wittgenstein (*Philosophical Investigations, IIxi*) begins his discussion of the duck-rabbit: 'Two uses of the word "see". The one: "What do you see there?"– "I see *this*" (and then a description, a drawing, a copy). The other: "I see a likeness between these two faces" – let the man I tell this to be seeing the faces as clearly as I do myself.' (*Philosophical Investigations*, translated by G.E.M. Anscombe, Oxford: Blackwell, p. 193).

Our skill at 'Mental rotation' is responsible for the widespread but mistaken belief that mirrors reverse left and right.
See Richard Gregory, '*Mirrors in Mind*' London: Penguin.

Swift's 'Big-Endians' and 'Little Endians' in 'Gulliver's Travels' fought over the correct way of opening an egg.
The influential 'two route' model of reading was put forward by Marshall, J. & Newcombe, F. (1973) 'Patterns of paralexia: A Psycholinguistic approach', *Journal of Psycholinguistic Research*, 2, 175–99. For a critical review see Shallice, T. (1988) *From Neuropsychology to Mental Structure* (Cambridge University Press).

Most of us, though perhaps not some kinds of Dyslexic, progress beyond letter-by-letter reading to the faster skill of reading by 'word shape.'
Given the obvious importance of word-shape it is surprising that there has been so much argument in the scientific literature about its role. Even until quite recently, it was thought that UPPER CASE TEXT could be read as quickly as lower case, and even that AlTeRnAtInG CaSe could be read as quickly as normal text. The problem with these early experiments is that they did not use sufficiently sensitive measures. Steven Dakin at UCL's Institute of Ophthalmology has put this subject on a new footing by using a sensitive psychophysical measure to measure performance. Observers had to decide whether simple syllogisms were true or false, when the propositions were presented very briefly, followed by a noise mask.

The shape of a word is defined by its length, by its pattern of descenders and ascenders, and by variations in density.
The idea that readers in Antiquity used only 'letter-by-letter' reading has been argued by John Mollon, who suggests that the invention of spaces was a decisive technological advantage allowing words to be read quickly by their shape. For Dyslexia and Italian see Paulesu, E. et al (2000) 'Dyslexia: cultural diversity and biological unity', *Science*, 291, 2165–7.

A different kind of dyslexia is sometimes seen in the neurological syndrome of 'parietal neglect', which may have afflicted the novelist Charles Dickens.
See McManus, I. C. (2002) 'Charles Dickens: a neglected diagnosis', *The Lancet*, 358, 2158–61. The Staplehurst derailment is described by L.T.C. Rolt in his classic *Red for Danger*, Pan Books (1986). There are two possible explanations for the permanent defect in visual awareness on one side of space experienced by Dickens and by Wollaston's anonymous friend. One is the complete loss of vision experienced by Inouye's patients, caused by damage to the primary visual map in the occipital cortex. The other is the 'neglect' syndrome (see chapter 11) and which is an incomplete visual awareness of one side of personal space associated with damage to the parietal lobe. Dickens's problem seems to have been mainly associated with reading, so it is unlikely to have been caused by damage to the primary visual area. The *Lancet* article argues that Dickens's symptoms are consistent with 'neglect dyslexia', caused by damage to the right parietal lobe affecting the left side of visual space. We shall never know with certainty whether this is the correct interpretation.

Dickens may have been suffering from the neurological condition called 'neglect dyslexia' associated with damage to the lower part of parietal lobe.

At the time of writing, the most recent book on neglect is Karnath, H.-O, Milner, A., & Vallar, G. (2002) *The Cognitive and Neural Bases of Spatial Neglect*, Oxford University Press. A brief and useful review is by Driver, J. & Jason Mattingley, J. (1998) 'Parietal neglect and visual awareness', *Nature Neuroscience*, 1998, 1, 17–22. For another useful review, containing the anecdote about make-up, see Fahle, M. (2002) 'Failures of visual stimulation: scotoma, Agnosia and Neglect', in Fahle, M. & Greenlee, M. (eds.), *Visual Neuropsychology*, Oxford University Press. For a general account of the role of the parietal cortex in perception see Colby, C. & Goldberg, M. (1992) 'Space and attention in parietal cortex,' *Ann. Rev. Neuroscience*, 233,10–49. The famous experiment on the Piazza de Duomo is in Bisiach, E. & Luzzanatti, C. (1978) 'Unilateral neglect of representational space', *Cortex*,14,129–33. See also Bisiach, E. (1993) 'Mental representation in unilateral neglect and related disorders: the twentieth Bartlett Lecture', *Quarterly Journal of Experimental Psychology*, A, 46, 435–61. The description of the problems in the Piazza of 'Signor Piazza' (not his real name) is taken from Beschin, N., Basso, A., & Sala, S. D. (2000) 'Perceiving left and imagining right', *Cortex*, 36, 401–14.

The explanation is unhelpful without a definition of attention.
William James was the brother of novelist Henry, and one of the few psychologists to appear in an important poem (Robert Lowell, *For the Union Dead*). For the relation between attention and neglect see Driver, J. (2001) 'A selective review of selective attention research from the past century', *British J. Psychology*, 92, 53–78.

11: Frames of Reference

By the 1870's the long task of finding out of which parts of the brain do what was well under way.
For an account of the Ferrier-Munk controversy see Glickstein, M. (1998) 'The Discovery of the Visual Cortex', *Scientific American*, 118–27

The problem of transforming frames of reference between different observers.
The quotation is from Colby, C. & Goldberg, M. (1999) 'Space and Attention in Parietal Cortex', *Annual Review of Neuroscience*, 22, 319–49. Other key articles on multiple maps are: Arbib, M. (1991) 'Interaction of multiple representations of space in the brain', in J. Paillard (ed.), *Brain and Space*, pp. 379–403, Oxford University Press; Jeannerod, M. et al (1965) 'Grasping objects: the cortical mechanisms of visuomotor transformation', *Trends in Neuroscience*, 18, 314–20

The simplest frame of reference for visual space is the eye itself.
The experiment on monkey eye–hand is reported by Snyder L. H. et al (2002) 'Eye-hand coordination: Saccades are faster when accompanied by a coordinated arm movement', *J. Neurophys.*, 87, 2279–86. The idea that any position on the retina is equivalent to the vector required to move the fovea to that point is what Hermann Lotze had in mind when he claimed that 'local sign' is nothing other than a feeling of effort required for an eye movement. The mechanics of moving the eye in its orbit with six sets of muscles is complicated, but luckily there is a very simple result. 'Donder's Law' states that the three dimensional position of the eye in the orbit depends only on the direction in which we are looking, and not on the previous history of eye movements. In other words, if I am looking at an object A and transfer my gaze to a different object B, the position of the eye in the orbit will be the same as if I had moved from A to C and from C to B. To some

extent movements of the arm show the same simplicity as those of the eye, as the reader can verify with another very cheap experiment. Try reaching for an object on a table in front of you, starting out from different initial positions of the arm on the table, and you will see that the position of the elbow and shoulder joint depends mainly on the position of the target you are reaching for, not on the starting position. However, Donder's Law for arm movements is not as exact as for movements of the eye, and it has been suggested that a more important principle is minimizing the amount of work that has to be done in making the movement.

The crude explanation is obvious – we retain some sort of mental image of the object's position in space.
For an account of 'efference copy' in relation to this problem see Merton, P. (1964) 'Human position sense and the sense of effort', *Symp. Soc. Exp. Biol.*, 18, 387–400. and Merton, P. (1961) 'The accuracy of directing the eyes and the hands in the dark', *Journal of Physiology*, 156, 555–77.

Against this, it could (and has been) argued that the colour in Dodge's experiment was too briefly presented to be perceived.
The subject of 'saccadic suppression' (as it is called) remains controversial. For the view that there is active suppression of visibility see Burr, D. C., Morgan, M. J., & Morrone, M. C. (1999) 'Saccadic suppression precedes visual motion analysis', *Curr Biol.*, 9(20), 1207–9; Burr, D. C., Morrone, C., & Ross, J. (1995) 'Selective suppression of the magnocellular visual pathway during saccadic eye movements', *Nature*, 371, 511–13. For the contrary view that objects remain visible if they are not blurred see Castet, E. & Masson, G. S. (2000) 'Motion perception during saccadic eye movements', *Nat. Neurosci.*, 3(2), 177–83.

Laboratory experiments have demonstrated this spatial distortion, and have even shown that the process of distortion starts in time slightly before the eye movement takes place.
The original experiments were by L. Matin. For more recent evidence see: Ross, J., Morrone, M. C., Goldberg, M. E., & Burr, D. C. (2001) 'Changes in visual perception at the time of saccades', *Trends Neurosci.*, 24(2), 113–21.

Another experiment shows what happens when the updating mechanism fails.
See the experiments on 'Eye Movements and Perception of Motion' in the Appendix.

A few simple experiments have taken us quite a long way towards understanding the complex transformations that happen to our spatial map when we move our eyes.
For the experiment on pointing in the dark see Henriques, D. Y. P. et al, (1998) 'Gaze-centered remapping of remembered visual space in an open-loop pointing task', *J. Neurosci.*,18, 1583–94. The experiment on pointing to a remembered sound source was carried out by Pouget, A. et al (2002) 'Multisensory spatial representations in eye-centered coordinates for reaching', *Cognition*, 83, B1–B11. Relevant to their conclusion that vision and sound share a common reference frame is the earlier experiment by Harris, C. S. (1963) 'Adaptation to displaced vision: visual, motor or proprioceptive change?', *Science*, 140, 812–13.

In another experiment, using 'virtual reality', observers saw a three-dimensional virtual world or 'workspace' in which they could move their arm.
Vetter, P., Goodbody, S., & Wolpert, D, (1999) 'Evidence for an eye-centered spherical representation of the visuomotor map', *J. Neurophys.*, 81, 935–9.

The parietal lobe is strategically placed ...
For the cell numbers and the fourfold increase in size of the cerebellum see Llinás, R. & Walton, K. D. (1990) 'Cerebellum' in Shepherd, G. M. (ed.), *The Synaptic Organisation of the Brain*, Oxford University Press. For connections between parietal lobe and pons – and thence cerebellum- see the now classic article by Glickstein, M. & May, J. G. (1982) 'Visual control of movement: the circuits which link visual to motion areas of the brain with special reference to the pons and cerebellum' in W. Neff (ed.), *Contributions to Sensory Physiology'* Vol 7 Academic Press, NY pp 103–45. See also Milner, A. D. & Goodale, M. A. (1995) *The Visual Brain in Action*, Oxford Universtity Press. There has been insufficient space in this book to consider the influence of the frontal lobes on movement: for this, see Passingham, R. (1993) *The Frontal Lobes and Voluntary Action*, Oxford University Press. Concerning the apocryphal window cleaner, I am not aware of any references in print, but the story was confidently told to us as undergraduates in Cambridge in the early 60's. Mitchell Glickstein has tried to trace the brain in question, but has found no trace of it (personal communication).

The answer is 'memory and planning'.
The scientific literature on LIP and the other parietal sub-division is dauntingly huge and complex. In compiling the very broad summary in this chapter I have found the following reviews indispensable: Andersen, R., Snyder, L., Li, C.-S., & Stricanne, B. (1993) 'Coordinate transformation in the representation of spatial information', *Current opinion in Neurobiology*, 3, 171–6; Baringa, M. (1999) 'The mapmaking Mind', *Science*, 285, 189–92; Colby, C., & Goldberg, M. (1999) 'Space and Attention in Parietal Cortex', *Annual Review of Neuroscience*, 22, 319–49; Snyder, L. (2000) 'Coordinate transformations for eye and arm movements in the brain', *Current Opinion in Neurobiology*, 10, 747–54; Xing, J., & Andersen, R. (2000) 'Models of the Posterior Parietal Cortex which perform multimodal integration and represent space in several coordinate frames', *Journal of Cognitive Neuroscience*, 12, 601–14.

Remapping is not an entirely automatic process.
See the review by Snyder (above), p. 748. Pursuit of 'snowflakes' is described by Ward, R., & Morgan, M. J. (1978) 'Perceptual effect of pursuit eye movements in the absence of a target' *Nature*, 274, 158–9.

There is an alternative explanation.
Klier, E., Wang, H. T., & Crawford, D. (2001) 'The superior colliculus encodes gaze command in retinal coordinates', *Nature Neuroscience*, 4, 627–32.

The arm may be another procrastinator.
Batista, A., et al (1999) 'Reach plans in eye-centered coordinates', *Science*, 285, 257–60.

We have assumed so far that vision provides the only information about the position of our arm in space.
For the experiment on the fake arm see Graziano, M.., Cooke, D., & Taylor, C. (2000)

'Coding the location of the arm by sight', *Science*, 290, 1782–6. The classic experiment on prisms and pointing to sounds was performed by Harris, C. S. (1963) op cit.

Sound also has to be put together with vision and touch.
For the mechanism guiding re-registration of the auditory map in owls see Hyde, P. & Knudsen, E. (2002) 'The optic tectum controls visually guided plasticity in the owl's auditory space map', *Nature*, 415, 73–6. This paper reports that if a small area in the visual map is destroyed, the corresponding area of the auditory map no longer shifts after adaptation to prisms. The crucial signal for transformation therefore seems to arise in the visual map.

The conclusion is that there are several maps of space in the brain.
The quotation about multiple maps is from the review by Colby, C. & Goldberg, M. (1999) 'Space and Attention in Parietal Cortex', *Annual Review of Neuroscience*, 22, 319–49.

12: Who Killed the Chauffeur?

In Raymond Chandler's novel The Big Sleep *(1939) Owen Taylor is the chauffeur for the Sternwood family.*
Chandler's letter to Hamish Hamilton from *Selected Letters of Raymond Chandler* (Frank McShane, ed., Macmillan, 1983) pp. 155–6. Taylor probably committed suicide after shooting the pornographer Geiger and finally seeing Carmen Sternwood, with whom he was in love, as the hopeless degenerate she was. One of the police at the pier scene points out that the car was driven hard and fast to the end of the pier. The tyre tracks were dead straight. Taylor's head wound is explained in a conversation between Marlow and small-time crook Joe Brody, who claims that he followed Taylor after he had shot Geiger and took from him the blackmail photographs of Carmen, after hitting Taylor with a sap. Brody is the only person who could plausibly have killed Taylor. His motive would have been to throw blame for Geiger's murder on Taylor, by putting the murder weapon in Taylor's car.

The failure of most readers to spot problems like Taylor's death could be put down to the complexity of plot and the fallibility of memory.
For continuity errors in *Citizen Kane* see <u>htpp:/www.movie-mistakes.com/</u>, and for further errors see <u>htpp:/erreursdefilms.free.fr/indexus/htm</u>. The *Farewell My Lovely* example is mentioned in a recent review, which gives many other examples (Levin, D. T. & Simons, D. J. (2000) 'Perceiving stability in a changing world: combining shots and integrating views in motion pictures and the real world', *Mediapsychology*, 2, 357–80).

Continuity blindness tells us that we take in less from our eyes than we think.
For further discussion see Dennett, D. (1991) *Consciousness Explained*, Allen Lane, The Penguin Press. See also O'Regan, K. & Noe, A. (2001) 'A sensorimotor account of vision and visual consciousness', *Behav. Brain Sci.*, 24, 955–75.

'Filling in' also happens at the 'blind spot'.
See Appendix for an experiment and further phenomena. For the debate on 'filling in' see Pessoa, L., Thompson, E., & Noe, A. (1998) 'Finding out about filling-in: a guide to perceptual completion for visual science and the philosophy of perception', *Behav. Brain*

Sci., 21(6), 723–48.; Ramachandran, V. S. & Gregory, R. L. (1991) 'Perceptual filling in of artificially induced scotomas in human vision', *Nature*, 350(6320), 699–702. Ramachandran & Gregory produced 'artificial blind-spots' in twinkling noise by reducing the intensity of points within a small area; this area rapidly becomes invisible like the natural blind spot, but more crucially, when the surrounding twinkling pattern is switched off, the previously blank area appears for a few brief moments to twinkle.

The challenge for psychologists, then, is to design experiments that distinguish between immediate perception and memory.
The question has a long history, going back to the experiments of Donald Broadbent in the '50s and '60s. If we listen to two different voices at the same time with stereo headphones it is quite easy to listen to one of them and to ignore the other. The 'rejected' message is hardly remembered at all, but how much of it was analysed at the time? If the 'rejected' message contains our own name, we tend to hear it, suggesting that some analysis was going on after all. For a very readable review of the 'early vs late' selection controversy see Pashler, H. E. (1998) *The Psychology of Attention*, Cambridge, Mass.: MIT Press.

Change blindness and the attentional blink are dramatic and entertaining phenomena.
For a recent review see O'Regan & Noe (op cit) and a forthcoming special issue of the *Journal of Vision* (2003).

Attention was memorably compared by the French Philosopher Maurice Merleau-Ponty to a searchlight.
The searchlight metaphor was used by the phenomenologist Maurice Merleau-Ponty, for whom it encapsulates what is wrong with Anglo-Saxon empiricism (*The Phenomenology of Perception*, London: Routledge, 1972), p. 26ff. For a later version, see Crick, F. (1984) 'Function of the thalamic reticular complex: the searchlight hypothesis', *Proceedings of the National Academy of Science*, 81, 4586–90. Merleau-Ponty was not one of the aliases used by de Selby, although their theories are sometimes similar. De Selby believed that the major problem the brain has to face is to dissipate the heat caused by thought. The savant advanced an interesting 'radiator theory' as an evolutionary explanation of baldness, pointing out that Men and Parrots are the only creatures who combine reason with developmental hair loss; but he was forced to withdraw this improbable conjecture after an outcry from Feminists. It is possible to see in this regrettable episode the origin of the savant's 'Engram Box', advertised as an 'Energy Efficient' aid to the formation of memories. See the article by Le Nie in *Certain considerations regarding the Power of Thought, Handbook of Neuroenergetics*, vol. XXI.

Results seemed to support the searchlight theory.
Beck, D. M. et al (2001) 'Neural correlates of change detection and change blindness', *Nature Neuroscience*, 4, 645–50. For a review of such studies see Rees, G. & Lavie, N. (2001) 'What can functional imaging tell us about the role of attention in visual awareness?', *Neuropsychologia*, 39,1343–53 and Rees, G. (2001) 'Neuroimaging of visual awareness in patients and normal subjects', *Current Opinion in Neurobiology*,11,150–56.

Another way of looking for the 'searchlight' is to record from single cells in monkeys when they are attending to a target.

Reynolds, J. H., Pasternak, T., & Desimone, R. (2000) 'Attention increases sensitivity of V4 neurons', *Neuron*, 26, 703–14.

Attention is about choosing between alternative courses of action.
The microstimulation experiment is reported by Moore, T. & Fallah, M. (2001) 'Control of eye movements and visual attention', *Proc. Nat. Acad. Sci. Am.*, 98,1273–6; Gardner, J. L. & Lisberger, S. G. (2002) 'Serial linkage of target selection for orienting and tracking eye movements', *Nature Neuroscience*, 5, 892–9. The comment is by Shadlen, M. (2002) 'Pursuing commitments', *Nature Neuroscience*, 5, 819–21.

13: Where is Fancy Bred?

Where is fancy bred?
The Merchant of Venice, Act 3, scene 2.

'Some times since it was imagined that deafness had been relieved by electrifying the patient...'
W. Watson, *Philosophical Transactions of the Royal Society*, 1751, 47, 202–11. For dreams and images in the blind see a review by Diego Kaski, *Perception*, in press. For the phenomenology of Charles Bonnet syndrome see Santhouse, A. M., Howard R. J. & Ffytche, D. H. (2000) *Brain*, 123, 2055–64.

Even stronger evidence is that blind people can see small electrical pulses applied directly to the brain itself.
The pioneering work was done by Brindley G. S. & Lewin, W. S. (1968) 'The sensations produced by electrical stimulation of the visual cortex', *J. Physiol.*, 196, 479–93. The case described here is based on the account by W.H. Dobelle of the Institut Dobelle AG Zurich. See *ASAIO Journal*, 2000, 46(1) 3–9. (ASAIO is the American Society of Artificial Internal Organs). It is not certain which cortical brain area is being stimulated by the electrode array. The distorted map of phosphenes on to external space does not correspond to what we would expect from the primary visual cortex (V1).

The Astronauts on Apollo 11 experienced flashes of light with their eyes closed.
See the Web site http://www.lbl.gov/Science-Articles/Archive/cornelius-tobias.
The 'Emmert's Law' experiment on phosphenes was done by Cowey, A. & Walsh, V. (2000) 'Magnetically-induced phosphenes in sighted, blind and blindsighted observers', *Neuroreport*, 11, 3269–73. For experiments on Emmert's Law see the Appendix.

'The cause of Sense is the Externall Body'.
Hobbes' target here is an alternative theory of vision apparently still being taught in the 'Universities of Christendome', which says that objects send little copies of themselves into the eye. 'I say not this as disapproving the use of Universities; but because I am to speak thereafter of their office in a Commonwealth, I must let you see on all occasions by the way, what things would be amended in them; amongst which the frequency of insignificant speech is one' (*Leviathan*, edited by C.B. Macpherson, Penguin Books 1968, chapter 1). It is curious that de Selby never comments on atmospheric perspective in his 'black air' theory of darkness. The obvious problem that we can see in the dark with the help of matches can be overcome by supposing that matches (and, indeed, perhaps,

torches) facilitate the passage of the little copies of objects through the otherwise murky atmosphere.

When we stimulate the striate cortex, the activity spreads to other areas of the occipital, temporal and parietal cortex, and eventually to the frontal lobe.
The experiments on single cells in V5/MT of conscious monkeys were reported by Newsome, W. T., Britten, K. H., & Movshon, J. A. (1989) 'Neuronal correlates of a perceptual decision', *Nature*, 341, 52–4.

Can it be cut by colour?
Zeki, S. et al (1999) 'The neurological basis of conscious color perception in a blind patient' *Proc. Nat. Acad. Sci. Am.*, 96(24), 14124–29. The patient PB, suffered an electric shock that led to vascular insufficiency, and became virtually blind, although he retained a capacity to see colours consciously. The fMRI results showed that, when he viewed and recognised colours, significant increases in activity were restricted mainly to V1-V2. The authors conclude 'that a partly defective color system operating on its own in a severely damaged brain is able to mediate a conscious experience of color in the virtually total absence of other visual abilities'. On the face of it, this result does not support the view that colour sensation happens exclusively in a special pre-striate area, but it is difficult to be precise when damage is so widespread. A further clue comes from 'colour synaesthetes' – people who experience colours when they hear or see. For 'colour organs' see htpp://rhythmiclight.com. The fMRI study is by Nunn J. A. et al (2002) 'Functional magnetic resonance imaging of synesthesia: activation of V4/V8 by spoken words', *Na. Neurosci*, 5(4), 371–5.

For many neuroscientists, fMRI finally cuts the Gordian knot.
For the spatial resolution of fMRI see Savoy, R. L. (2003) 'Imaging the Visual Brain', in M.A. Arbib (ed.), *The Handbook of Brain Theory and Neural Networks*, second Edition, Cambridge, Mass.: MIT Press.

14: Unconscious Perception

Patients with complete damage of the primary visual cortex (V1) are blind, in the ordinary and legal sense of the term.
But they do have connections from the (intact) retina to other parts of the brain. Some nerve fibres in the optic nerve apparently get routed to V5 without passing through V1. For a review and account of the 'retrograde degeneration' experiment see Cowey, A. & Stoerig, P. (1991) 'The neurobiology of blindsight', *Trends Neurosci.*,14,140–45. Functional imaging studies have shown that the 'motion area' V5 responds to moving stimuli in the blind part of the visual field: see Zeki, S. (1998) 'Parallel processing, asynchronous perception, and a distributed system of consciousness in vision', *Neuroscientist*, 4, 365–72. One study has reported activity in V5 of a hemianopic patient without conscious awareness (Goebel, R. et al (2001) 'Sustained extrastriate cortical activation without visual awareness revealed by fMRI studies of hemianopic patients', *Vision Res*, 41, 1459–74.

The British Army doctor G. Riddoch treated soldiers with head injuries during the First World War...
Riddoch, G. (1917) 'Dissociation of visual perceptions due to occipital injuries, with

especial reference to appreciation of movement', *Brain*, 40,15–57., cited by Cowey, A. & Azzopardi, P. (2001) 'Is Blindsight motion blind?', in De Gelder, B., De Haan, E., & Heywood, C. (eds.), *Out of Mind: Varieties of Unconscious Experience*, Oxford University Press. Residual vision was described by Poeppel, E., Held, R. & Frost, D. (1973) 'Residual visual function after brain wounds involving the central visual pathways in man', *Nature*, 243, 295–6., and 'blindsight' by Weiskrantz, L. et al (1974) 'Visual capacity in hemianopic field following a restricted occipital ablation' , *Brain*, 97, 709–28. See also Weiskrantz, L. (1986) *Blindsight: a case study and its implications*, Oxford University Press,. and De Gelder, B., De Haan, E., & Heywood., C. (2001, op cit). For a critical review of the latter see Morgan, M. J. (2002) 'Detecting the wrong signals?', *Trends in Cognitive Neuroscience*, 6, 443–44.

Many thousands of words have been written on this topic, some of them quite acrimonious.
See the review by Semir Zeki of the book *Out of Mind* in *The Times Higher Education Supplement*, 29 March 2002, and replies by the authors on the 12 and 19 April.

The sensation of the speck that bore the King was uncertain, as is typical of weak or 'noisy' sensation.
It is fair to point out that many cognitive psychologists disagree with my analysis here. They reject Signal Detection Theory as an account of perception, and think of perception as an all-or-none process. Unconscious perception means just that: there was no mental experience *at all* corresponding to the event in question, but it subsequently influences behaviour. My answer to that is a question: how could you ever prove that there was no mental experience *at all* at the time of the event? Merely talking to the person is insufficient: the signal has already been filtered by all the brain mechanisms required for language. The only way to be sure would be to show that the event in question had no effect at all *on the brain*. But then it could have no effect on behaviour!

In an fMRI experiment using this logic, observers were tested in the 'repetition priming' experiment described earlier.
Dehaene, S. et al. (2001) 'Cerebral mechanisms of work masking and repetition priming', *Nature Neuroscience*, 2001, 4, 752–8. See also the commentary by Rees in the same issue of the journal (678–80), on which my own inferences from the experiment are largely based.

15: The Secretion Theory of Consciousness

'When Cabanis said that thought was a function of the brain, in the same sense as bile secretion is a function of the liver, he blundered philosophically'...
Huxley goes on to say: 'But in the mathematical sense of the word 'function' thought may be a function of the brain.' He means that there is a one-to-one correspondence (mapping) between brain states and thoughts, such that no single brain state corresponds to more than one thought. Note that the mathematical definition of a function does not exclude the possibility that different brain states correspond to the same thought. If a set of numbers **A** is a function of a different set **B**, then different numbers in **A** must correspond to different numbers in **B**. But different numbers in **B** are allowed by the definition of a function to correspond to the same numbers in **A**. Tan(x) is a function, but the inverse $tan^{-1}(x)$ is not, despite the claims of pocket calculators.

To be sure, there are small differences in microscopic structure across the cortex.
For the uniformity hypothesis that the cortex is pretty much the same everywhere see Douglas, R. J. & Martin, K. A. C. (1990) 'Neocortex', in G. M Shephard (ed.), *The Synaptic Organisation of the Brain*, Oxford University Press, pp. 389–438. As they say 'If this view is correct, it then leads to the fascinating question of how the functional differences between the areas arise if they have the same basic microcircuitry.'

In other words, we see colour when our brain classifies part of the retinal image as coming from a surface of a particular type.
For a clinical account of auditory-seeing see Jacobs, L., Karpik, A., & Bozian, D. (1981) 'Auditory-visual synaesthesia', *Archives of Neurology*, 38, 211–16.

Like collectors of rare stamps, neuroscientists looking for conscious brain mechanisms hope that they will be few in number.
Crick, F. & Koch, C. (1995) 'Are we aware of activity in primary visual cortex?', *Nature*, 375,121–3.

Rivalry is illustrated by the images composed of coloured rings . . .
Treisman, A. (1962) 'Binocular rivalry and stereoscopic depth perception', *Quart. J. Exp. Psychol.*, 14, 23–37.

Rivalry can also be seen in the textures illustrated in Figure 15.2.
The experiment with crossed images in the two eyes was done by Kolb, F. C. & Braun, J. (1995) 'Blindsight in normal observers', *Nature*, 377, 336–8., and followed up by Morgan, M. J., Mason, A., & Solomon, J. A. (1997) 'Blindsight in normal observers', *Nature*, 385, 401–2.

Rivalry may seem to argue that V1 does, after all, make a 'direct contribution' to awareness.
For thoughts on the Diaz-Caneja figure see Ngo, T. T. et al (2000) 'Binocular rivalry and perceptual coherence', *Curr. Biol.*,10, R134–R136., where the experiment was successfully repeated with black-white stimuli. For a translation of the original paper see htpp://psy.otago.ac.nz/br-Djtrans.html.

These arguments are complicated, and it is tempting once again to cut the Gordian knot with brain imaging.
For Darwin's experiments see Simons, P. (1992) 'The secret feelings of plants', *New Scientist*, 17 Oct. The story of Darwin's gardener is related in the audio commentary by David Attenborough to the tour of Down House (highly recommended). Bose's experiments are related by Diaz-Caneja (see previous note).

Bose's idea that rivalry starts in the eye has had no support from later research.
For a review of the evidence up to 1989 see section 8.8 of Howard & Rogers (1995, op cit). The fMRI experiment with different contrast patterns was reported by Polonsky, A. et al (2000) 'Neuronal activity in human primary cortex correlates with perception during binocular rivalry', *Nat. Neurosci.*, 3, 1153–9. Note that the correlation was also found in V2, V3 and V4, so the results do not rule out a contribution of 'higher' centres to rivalry. They only contradict the idea that V1 is not involved.

Despite this apparently conclusive evidence for rivalry in V1, other experiments disagree.

See Ngo, T. T. et al. (2000) 'Binocular rivalry and perceptual coherence', *Curr Biol*,10, R134–R136;.Leopold, D. A. & Logothetis, N. (1999) 'Multistable phenomena: changing views in perception', *Trends Cogn. Sci.*, 3, 254–64. The experiment on rivalry in monkeys is reported in Leopold, D. A. & Logothetis, N. (1996) 'Activity changes in early visual cortex reflect monkey's percepts during binocular rivalry', *Nature*, 379, 549–53.

Sauce for the goose is sauce for the gander.

See Thompson, K. G. & Schall, J. D. (1999) 'The detection of visual signals by macaque frontal eye fields during rivalry', *Nat. Neurosci.*, 2, 283–8. See also the 'News and Views' in the same issue by J. Assad. Monkeys were trained to move their eyes to a rapidly flashed target in the periphery of their vision. The target could be flashed at any one of eight points on an imaginary circle at the monkey's point of regard. Just after the target flashed it was followed by a 'mask' consisting of flashes at every one of the eight possible target positions. For human observers, the mask makes the target very difficult to see, provided the time interval between target flash and mask is sufficiently small (less than about 30 thousandths of a second). This interval was shortened until the monkeys made eye movements to the target on only about 50 per cent of the occasions when the target was actually present. Now, it had been previously established that nerve cells in an area of the monkey's frontal cortex known as the 'frontal eye fields' tended to fire only when a target was flashed within its 'receptive field.' In other words, a given cell might respond when a target was flashed in the 3 o'clock position but not when the target was flashed in the 6 o'clock position. The crucial question was what would happen to the cell when the target was flashed in the 3 o'clock position but followed by a mask to make it visible on only 50 per cent of the trials. If the cell is involved in conscious detection we expect it to fire only on trials when the monkey detected the target. In fact, the cell responded on all trials, irrespective of whether the monkey made an eye movement or not. We cannot conclude from this that cells in the frontal eye fields make no contribution to conscious experience. The firing of the '3 o'clock' cell may well have been involved in the monkey's experiencing a target in the 3 o'clock position. The problem is that the 'mask' will almost certainly have caused cells in the other positions around the clock to respond as well. The monkey, or some part of the monkey's brain, has to decide whether the activity in the 3 o'clock cell exceeds the activity of other cells to a point where the presence of a target in the 3 o'clock position can be inferred. The comparison of the outputs of cells is a process bedevilled by 'noise', so there will be many trials when the monkey makes a mistake and decides not to respond. This does not necessarily mean that there was no experience corresponding to the firing of the '3 o'clock' cell on trials when the monkey decided not to respond. When the watchers saw King Arthur's burial ship 'go on and on and vanish into light' there would have come a time when they finally decided that the boat was invisible. Some cells in the brain activated by the image of the boat might nonetheless have still been active. But so would many other cells. It is impossible to infer the contents of consciousness from the activity of a single nerve cell, and this argument applies as much to the primary visual cortex as it does to the supposedly 'higher' centre of the frontal eye fields.

16: Into the Mill

The map in the primary visual cortex (V1) has become the battlefield for this new philosophical conflict.

See Crick, F. & Koch, C. (2003) 'A framework for consciousness', *Nat. Neurosci.*, 6(2), 119–26. The experiment on the 'waterfall effect' was by Lehmkuhle, S. W. & Fox, R. (1975) 'Effect of binocular rivalry suppression on the motion after-effect, *Vision Res.*, 15, 855–9.. It would be difficult to confine presentation of the moving stimulus to periods when it was invisible. What Lehmkuhle & Fox actually did was to measure the strength (duration) of the waterfall effect as a function of the length of time it was presented to the eye, versus the length of time it was visible in a rivalry situation. They found that time on the retina was more important than the time for which the stimulus was seen. See also Blake, R. & Fox, R. (1974) 'Adaptation to invisible gratings and the site of binocular rivalry suppression', *Nature*, 249, 488–90.

If crowding is severe, observers cannot tell whether a target line is tilted horizontally (–) or vertically (|), when it is surrounded by other tilted lines.

For the experiment on adaptation to 'crowded' lines and for references to the causes of adaptation itself see He, S., Cavanagh, P., & Intriligator, J. (1996) 'Attentional resolution and the locus of visual awareness', *Nature*, 383, 334–7. Their experiment used patches of windowed sine-wave gratings rather than single lines. For other experiments showing behavioural effects of 'invisible' patterns see MacLeod, D. I. A. & He, S. (1992) 'Visible flicker from invisible patterns', *Nature*, 362, 256–8;. Smallman, H. et al (1996) 'Fine-grain of the neural representation of human spatial vision', *J. Neurosci.*,16,1852–9. For an experiment suggesting that observers still have access to 'crowded lines' for texture perception see Parkes, L. et al (2001) *Nature Neuroscience*, 4, 739–44.

So the evidence to convict V1 of insentience is still inconclusive.

For the detection experiment see Azzopari, P. & Cowey, A. (1997) 'Is blindsight like normal, near-threshold vision?', *Proc. Natl. Acad. Sci.*, 94,14190–4., and comments by Morgan, M. J. (2002) 'Detecting the wrong signals?', *Trends Cog. Neurosci.*, 6443–4.

Another line of attack on the problem of GY's awareness has been to see if he can 'match' the appearance of images in his 'blind' field of vision to other images in his normal field.

See Stoerig, P. & Barth, E. (2001) 'Low-level phenomenal vision despite unilateral destruction of primary visual cortex', *Conscious. Cogn.*, 10, 574–87. For the unilateral colour-blind case see MacLeod, D. I.A. & Lennie, P. (1976) 'Red-green blindness confined to one eye', *Vision Res.*, 16, 691–702.

A recent idea, from two neuropsychologists Milner and Goodale, is that visual awareness is associated with the 'ventral pathway' alone.

Milner, A. D. & Goodale, M. A. (1995) *The Visual Brain in Action*, Oxford University Press. The idea of separate pathways for action and shape was proposed by Glickstein, M. & May, J. G. (1982) 'Visual control of movement: the circuits which link visual to motion areas of the brain with special reference to the pons and cerebellum', *Contributions to Sensory Physiology*, vol 7.,103–45. At roughly the same time a similar dichotomy was proposed by Ungerleider, L. G. & Mishkin, M. (1982) 'Two cortical visual systems', in Ingle, D. J., Goodale, M. A., & Mansfield, R. J. W. (eds.) *Analysis of Visual*

Behaviour, Cambridge Mass.: MIT Press, pp. 383–400. (see also Mishkin, M., Ungerledier, L. A., & Macko, K. A. (1983) 'Object vision and spatial vision: two cortical pathways', *Trends in Neuroscience*, 6, 414–17.) The two pathways were called the 'what' and the 'where.' Even earlier, work on the hamster led to the idea that there were 'two visual systems', one for locating objects and the other for identifying them: Schneider, G. E. (1969) 'Two visual systems: brain mechanisms for localisation and discrimination are dissociated by tectal and cortical lesions', *Science*, 163, 895–902.

Another problem with the automaton theory comes from a brain imaging study of 'neglect'.
For a review of the evidence on this point see Rees, G. (2001) 'Neuroimaging of visual awareness in patients and normal subjects', *Current Opinion in Neurobiology*, 11,150–56.

Conclusion: The Search for the Grail

Against this, opponents of 'strong AI' say that a digital computer is merely a number cruncher, programmed by a human operator to simulate something else.
The argument has been put with particular force by John Searle in his metaphor of the 'Chinese Room' (Searle, J. (1980) 'Minds, Brains, and Programs', *Behavioral and Brain Sciences*, 3, 417–457). Daniel Dennett ('Consciousness Explained') criticises the 'Chinese Room' as unrealistic. A computer that was realistically able to translate English into Chinese would have to know what the symbols meant. For the pros and cons see the 'Internet Encyclopaedia of Philosophy' at
http://www.utm.edu/research/iep/c/chinese.htm

Appendix A

Demonstrations

The following demonstrations and experiments can all be performed at home without special apparatus.

The Pinhole Pupil (Chapter 1). Use a needle to punch a clean round hole in a sheet of stiff paper.

1. *Glickstein's Experiment*: Hold the pinhole in front of one eye while looking in a mirror and observe the size of the pupil in the uncovered eye. When the pinhole is taken away from the eye the pupil of the other eye contracts; when the pinhole is restored the pupil expands. Note that this happens in the uncovered eye. You have observed the 'consensual response of the pupils'. In other words, the two pupils always respond in the same way. The reason is that they are controlled by the same computer in the midbrain, which averages the light in the two eyes. You cannot directly observe the size of the pupil in the eye behind the pinhole, but you can see it indirectly by the following experiment. Place the pinhole in front of the left eye and note the size of the circle you see through it. Now place your hand in front of the right eye. The size of the circle seen through the pinhole gets larger. Remove your hand from the right eye and the circle gets smaller. The reason is that the size of the circle is determined by the size of the pupil. When the right eye is covered the average light from the two eyes is reduced so the pupils expand, thus enlarging the circle on the retina.
2. *Depth of field*. Observe that you can read text through a pinhole from a distance of only a few inches without its becoming blurred. (However, the page must be well illuminated). The explanation is that without the pinhole the text is blurred by rays that are permitted

by the natural pupil to pass through the outer part of the lens; these are not brought to a point of focus so they form a 'blur circle'. The pinhole prevents these marginal rays from reaching the retina.

The Pulfrich effect (Chapter 5). Set a pendulum (or equivalent such as a plumb line) swinging from left to right and examine it with a sunglass lens in front of the left eye (both eyes must be open). The pendulum will appear to swing in a clockwise ellipse. If the lens is in front of the right eye the direction of swing will be reversed. Look at objects moving on a TV in the same way. The TV will become three-dimensional. The effect is caused by a delay in transmitting the signal from the darker eye, which causes the covered eye to see objects later in time, and thus at an earlier point on their trajectory. The difference in apparent position between the two eyes is interpreted by the brain as a depth effect (see Chapter 4). For further explanation see the article on the Pulfrich effect in *The Oxford Companion to the Mind*, Edited by R.L. Gregory.

Eye Movements and Perception of Motion (Chapter 11). The curious incident of the nocturnal dog in *The Memoirs of Sherlock Holmes* was that it did nothing. Similarly curious is the absence of a perception of motion when we move our eyes. The image moves on the retina so why do we not see it as moving? The 'corollary discharge' theory says that the brain keeps a record of its instructions to the eye movement muscles and uses this to predict the expected amount of movement on the retina. If the prediction is correct, no movement is seen. Several phenomena follow from the theory. (1) If the eye is displaced by gentle pressure from the finger against the lower eyelid, the world should appear to move. The brain has no record of sending instructions to the eye movement muscles, so the movement of the retinal image is unanticipated. (2) If we form an afterimage on the retina (see Emmert's Law below for instructions on how to do this) and make voluntary eye movements in the dark, the afterimage will appear to move, but (3) if we move the eye by finger pressure in the dark, the afterimage will appear stationary.

The Blind Spot and other experiments on 'filling in' (Chapter 12). To see the blind spot, take a blank sheet of white paper and draw a small spot in the centre; then a cross two inches to the left. Close the right eye, and look steadily through the left eye at the paper held about one hand's length away from the eye, and note the appearance of the cross. As the paper is moved slowly away from or towards the eye, there should be a position at which the cross completely disappears. It has fallen in the 'blind spot'.

Other cases in which stimuli fade from consciousness are 'Troxler Fading' and 'Motion-Induced blindness. Troxler fading refers to the disappearance of small objects from peripheral vision if we hold steady fixation. For example, if we look steadily at one spot on a dirty window pane, the other spots fade out one by one like the stars at sunrise, the fainter Pleiades disappearing before their neighbour, the brighter Aldeberan. Troxler fading is presumably related to the fact that images fixed on the eye, like the afterimage of a photographic flash, fade rapidly from consciousness unless we blink to bring them back. Nerve cells in the retina also have this property, so perhaps Troxler fading arises there, or in the visual cortex. The connection between Troxler fading and the blind spot may be that in both cases we cease to see an object in the visual field when there are no sensory signals to tell us that it is there.

Even more dramatic than Troxler fading is the case of 'motion induced blindness', which can be seen at http://www.weizmann.ac.il/home/masagi/MIB/mib-basic.html. Three small yellow squares on a TV monitor are embedded in a swirling snowstorm of randomly moving blue dots. After only a few seconds the yellow squares disappear entirely from consciousness. The disappearance is unmistakable and astonishing. It is not identical to Troxler fading, because it happens much too quickly, and because it persists even if the image of the yellow squares on the retina is moved by tracking the little blue dots with the eyes. Somehow, the moving blue dots are wiping the static yellow squares from consciousness. It is impossible to see the effect and to believe that it is due to memory failure. The yellow squares disappear, and that's that. Perhaps the explanation is that when tracking moving objects we have to ignore the blurred image of the stationary background. Note how very hard it is to read a line of print if one concentrates on the tip of a pencil moving over it.

Emmert's Law (Chapter 13). Stare for a few seconds at an incandescent light bulb to produce an 'afterimage' on the retina, or look at the flash when your photograph is being taken. The afterimage fades rapidly, but can be restored by blinking. It will look like a black spot, sometimes surrounded by intensely saturated rings. Look at a nearby surface like the hand and the afterimage will seem to be superimposed on it. Note the apparent size. Now look at a more distant object, like a house outside the window. Again, the afterimage will appear superimposed, but will now seem much larger. The usual explanation for this is 'size constancy' – objects project smaller images on the retina if they are more distant, and the brain compensates. This, of course, is a name for the phenomenon, not a mechanism. One possibility is that we cannot escape judging the size of objects in relation to their surroundings. The distant afterimage covers a house; the nearby afterimage covers only the hand, and is therefore seen as smaller.

Leakage of sensations (Chapter 15). It is not easy to demonstrate 'leakage' of sensations from one sense organ to another. But accidental leakage from one colour pathway to another is much easier to observe. The great Czech physiologist Purkinje described 'blue arcs' that are seen at night when there is a small-ish bright red object in the visual field. Emanating from the object in wide arcs and ending at the 'blind spot' are intensely-saturated but evanescent violet streaks. The 'blue arcs of Purkinje', as they are called, are especially obvious around car brake-lights at night. Yellow sodium lights can substitute for car brake lights. A torch covered with a deep red cellophane is an excellent tool for experimenting. Look at the torch in a completely dark room, and you should see the blue arcs. Drawings of the blue arcs by an experienced observer correspond exactly to the route of the nerve fibres coursing from the image of the stimulating light to the 'blind spot' where they exit the eye to form the optic nerve. Somehow, the electrical impulses flowing along the nerve fibres must be leaking out and stimulating either the 'blue cones' directly, or the nerve cells to which they are connected. Since the brain knows only that the 'blue' cells are active, not what caused them to become active, we experience a blue sensation. This is the logical essence of a 'leakage' explanation. It is related to the late William Rushton's 'Principle of Invariance', which states that once a cone has absorbed a particle of energy, it loses all information about its wavelength. The 'blue arcs' are caused either by leakage along undiscovered nerve connections, or by direct leakage of current from the less-than-perfectly insulated optic nerve fibres. The mechanism is one of the remaining mysteries in the science of the retina.

Appendix B

Statement on animal experimentation

An interesting suggestion is that all doctor's surgeries and hospital waiting rooms should contain a prominent sign stating that no drugs will be prescribed unless they have been first tested on animals; and that wherever possible, new surgical procedures such as hip replacement have been practised on pigs. In a similar vein, any book, like this one, which describes our present state of knowledge of the brain should state honestly and clearly that this knowledge would not have been acquired without experiments on animals. Some opponents of animal experimentation will say that such experiments can be replaced by 'non-invasive' methods such as purely psychological observations and by functional brain imaging. This is similar to the argument that all drugs tests can be done in tissue culture, and just as mistaken. No competent scientist supports the idea that all drug tests could be done *in vitro*. Similarly, we would know nothing about nerve cells and their receptive fields without experiments on squid, cats and monkeys. As for the idea that functional brain imaging can replace animal experimentation in Neuroscience, the reader will be able to judge after reading this book. Functional imaging can tell us the location of some of the analogue computers that go to make up our brain, but does not come remotely near to telling us how these computers work.

Obviously, this does not mean that any experiments are justified by our curiosity. There are limits beyond which no sane individual will go. Different people would draw the line in different places, so it is for the public – through their political representatives – to decide where the line of legality should be drawn. I do not do any animal experiments myself, and therefore cannot be said to have any vested interest in the matter. I used to have a Home Office Licence to experiment with rats but became sentimental about them and ended up keeping rats as pets at home. (Oddly, the protesters outside Huntingdon Life Sciences have nothing to say about the millions of highly intelligent and inquisitive rats who are of necessity poisoned and gassed in our sewers each year.) If I did still work on animals I think I would draw my own line somewhere about the point where monkeys are deliberately injected with heroin to study the mechanisms of addiction. There is, arguably, something perverse about visiting our self-inflicted misfortunes on an animal with a similar brain to our own. Some scientists would clearly think differently, but this should be a matter of informed public debate, not a reason for vituperation – and still less, for violence.

If we accept the view that all life has value, most people would agree that animal life should be sacrificed only if there is some long term goal of relieving human (and animal) suffering. I submit that understanding how our brain works is clearly such a goal. This is based on first-hand experience. I grew up in the grounds of an old-style Psychiatric Hospital where my father was Medical Superintendent, and observed the nightmare of schizophrenia before there were any anti-psychotic drugs to control it. No film or play that I have seen about schizophrenia comes even close to revealing the true horror of the affliction before there was effective medication to control it. But present anti-psychotic drugs are only the beginning; they have undesirable side effects, and we still do not know the reason why the wiring of the brain goes wrong in adolescent schizophrenics. Nor do we know why certain cells degenerated in the brain of Mervyn Peake, making it impossible for him to complete the *Gormenghast* trilogy. But we will know, through experiments on animals, and one day Parkinsonism will be preventable. One day, also, Age-Related Macular Degeneration, the commonest cause of blindness in industrialised countries, may be cured – perhaps by implants, perhaps by gene therapy, perhaps by some other method undreamed of at present: but never without animal experiments. For example, designing a silicon replacement for the retina requires accurate knowledge about the mechanisms of seeing, based on animal experimentation.

Some pro-vivisectionists argue that opponents of animal experimentation have no right to use medical advances based on animals; and that they should sign a statement to this effect. This is even sillier than the idea that pacifists have no right to enjoy the benefits of Hitler's defeat and should therefore be placed in concentration camps. However, a weaker version is, I think arguable: opponents of animal experimentation in Neuroscience should be willing to explain to the relative of a person suffering from Alzheimer's or from Schizophrenia why they are trying to prevent fundamental science that will find the cause of these diseases.

Index